LIFE
AFTER
CANCER

2

LIFE
AFTER
CANCER

Ann Kent

WARD LOCK

A WARD LOCK BOOK
First published in the UK 1996
by Ward Lock
Wellington House
125 Strand
LONDON WC2R OBB

A Cassell Imprint

Distributed in the United States by Sterling Publishing Co., Inc.
387 Park Avenue South, New York, NY 10016-8810

Distributed in Australia by Capricorn Link (Australia) Pty Ltd
2/13 Carrington Road, Castle Hill NSW 2154

A British Library Cataloguing in Publication Data block for
this book may be obtained from the British Library

ISBN 0 7063 7458 4
Printed and bound in Finland

CONTENTS

FOREWORD

WHY ME? WHAT SHOULD I DO NEXT? How do I tell my friends? How do I cope with the system? This is an unusual book that provides answers to just these sorts of questions. Written by an experienced medical journalist, it covers a wide range of problems encountered by cancer patients, their friends and families. It does not pretend to be a cancer textbook: there are plenty of those around, whether for patients, general practitioners or specialists.

One in three of us alive today will develop cancer, but by the year 2020 the figure will be one in two because of changes in the age distribution of the population. So inevitably, we are all going to need the information in this book, whether for ourselves or for a loved one. Here you can find straightforward, sensible and yet sensitive advice on issues as diverse as getting back to work, sexual problems, overcoming stress, fear and anger, taking a positive approach, complementary therapies and finding the best medical care.

Despite all the information available on cancer, it is tough steering a path through the myriad of problems that confront a patient today. From the moment the diagnosis is confirmed, a series of decisions need to be made that require careful thought. Many of these have nothing to do with the technology of cancer treatment.

Ann uses examples from real life, and pulls no punches with her anecdotes. Unlike the evangelical stories of many cranky alternative therapies, where cancer can always be beaten by following a particular recipe, this book rings true. Believe me, if there were a wonder cure – however bizarre, conventional or alternative – we would all be using it. So an odyssey in search of a magic bullet is unlikely to prove fruitful.

The most powerful message for cancer patients is the need to avoid being emotionally engulfed by the disease. There is much one can do to help oneself here, with or without professional help. Relationships with friends and family may become altered. Unpredictable reactions are common, varying from very negative attitudes through to jealousy from children about the increased attention a parent is getting. Above all, adopting a positive approach requires a combination of self-will, determination and knowledge.

Although there are no maps provided for the cancer journey, this is an excellent and very readable guidebook.

Karol Sikora
Professor of Clinical Oncology, Hammersmith Hospital, and Deputy Director of Clinical Research, Imperial Cancer Research Fund, London.

INTRODUCTION

EACH YEAR MORE THAN A QUARTER OF A MILLION UK citizens will be told they have cancer. In the US, the figure is 1.25 million. For most of those people life will never be the same again.

The diagnosis of a potentially fatal illness unsettles all our plans for the future, and forces us to confront our own mortality. Yet many people do not begin to deal with the implications of their illness until they are released from the protective cocoon of the hospital. After a few weeks or months of treatment, the patient is discharged and told he or she can resume work and live as before. The days of grapes and flowers and sympathy are over, and the rest of the world wants to forget, and wants the person with cancer to forget as well. If you are in this situation, you may feel depressed, helpless and convinced your life is no longer under your control.

After reading the accounts of the cancer patients interviewed in this book, you may think you could never be as brave, or as stoical, or as philosophical. In fact, these interviews came easily and simply. Everyone I spoke to had a story to tell, and insights to offer. All were marked by their experiences, but some had come to the remarkable conclusion that cancer had actually improved their lives.

I had originally intended to interview all the top cancer specialists to canvass their views on survival. But in the end, it was the people who had experienced cancer who shaped and guided the book. They generously shared their painful and positive experiences, even though in everyday life many of them have now put their cancers on the back burner. I would like to dedicate the book to: Sylvia Bone, Kevin Brailsford, John Harrison, Sally Harrison, Renée Hesketh, Anne Johnson, Tony Johnson, Debbie Jones, Samantha Jones, Margaret Knight, Jim

Lain, Jane Oakley, Jeanette Pearson, George Turner, Jean Walker, Danny Wells and Sharon Willmott.

I would also like to thank everyone at the Imperial Cancer Research Fund for more than a decade of information, guidance and support; BACUP (the British Association of Cancer-United Patients) for its patient-friendly information; the Cancer Research Campaign, CancerLink, the Disability Alliance, the American Cancer Society, the National Cancer Alliance, Dr Maurice Slevin, Dr Amanda Ramirez, Prof. Karol Sikora, Kathleen Sheridan, Simon Darnley and countless other medical experts who have allowed their brains to be picked in the last couple of years.

CHAPTER 1

LIFE OUTSIDE THE HOSPITAL

*What matters is not whether we live or die,
because we all die. What matters is what
happens in the middle.*

DR MAURICE SLEVIN,
CANCER PHYSICIAN AND CHAIRMAN OF BACUP

WHY YOU FEEL THE WAY YOU DO

Having cancer is a lonely experience. However caring and concerned your friends and family may be, they cannot know how it feels to have cancer.

Most of us take our health for granted. A cancer diagnosis not only unsettles our sense of well-being, but all our certainties about the future. Even if you went through months suspecting that you might have cancer, you are likely to be shocked when the diagnosis is made. None of your previous experience is any help as you face this new situation.

Cancer can leave you in a limbo, no longer confident enough to plan your garden, holiday, pension scheme or career. It can also lead you to change totally your priorities in life – and often your lifestyle as well. Now the first wave of treatment is over, you will wonder whether it will be weeks or months or years before you feel normal again.

A recent study of women with cervical cancer found that two years after their treatment, nearly half still felt tired, lethargic and depressed. Doctors are currently trying to find ways of relieving such high levels of unhappiness. People with cancer cannot afford to wait for the results of this research. They will want to make sure they are in the second half of the group – the ones who regain their happiness and peace of mind after treatment.

We all vary in the way we react to a cancer diagnosis. For some people there is an immediate outpouring of grief. Others will be shocked and numb. Some people become furiously angry with their doctors for real or imagined failures in diagnosis and treatment, or they will demand to know 'why me?'. Others – the ones for whom control is most important – will not allow themselves to express any feelings at all. They may seem to sail through their hospital treatment, only to become severely depressed many months later. Cancer is a journey without maps, no matter how much you know about health and medicine.

Dr Maurice Slevin explains: 'I usually tell people that they are likely to be depressed when their treatment finishes, but they are always surprised when it happens. They realize how dependent they have become on the regular visits to the hospital, and how the treatment, however difficult, adds structure and security to their lives. For many people this is a time of introspection when they try to sort out the new meaning of their lives in a new world.'

It is natural to feel lost and vulnerable while the confident 'experts' discuss your case. Shock turns some people deaf during consultations with their doctor. Later on the specialist will say, 'But I told you about that' while the patient looks blank and helpless. This is normal too.

Some hospitals now tape-record consultations for their patients. Otherwise, there is no reason why a patient cannot make his or her own recording of the conversation. Some doctors may find this threatening, unless you explain your reasons, i.e. that you do not want to miss out on important information.

The diagnosis of cancer can take away the feeling of personal control that we all need to get through our lives. But often it is the little things that cause the most grief.

Most doctors now realize the need to give patients information about what they face but sometimes routine problems are not mentioned. You can come through major surgery and then be reduced to tears because no one warned that your wound might fill with fluid, or because no one told you that Dr X does things differently from Dr Y, or because your appointment has been put back or moved forward by a week. Because of your loss of control, you may find you lose your temper easily. Some people focus their anger on their hospital doctors, the messengers who brought them the original bad news about their cancers.

Once your operation scars have faded you may be raring to go back to work. However, many people are amazed and disillusioned to find they are unable to concentrate when they return to their jobs – or that even a routine day in the office exhausts them.

All of these initial reactions and any combination of them are normal. Problems will only arise if you get stuck at this stage of your recovery, so that you continue to be shocked, angry or depressed during the months when your body and spirits should be starting to heal.

When newspapers and magazines describe people with cancer, the focus is usually on the treatment, or on whether they have received the 'all clear' five years after the treatment has finished. The vital months or years in between are seldom mentioned, and yet healing at this time is as vital as anything that occurs in hospital.

Cancer has many survivors. The difference between the numbers of people diagnosed with the disease each year (300,000) and the numbers who die of it (140,000) is 160,000. In the US, 1,252,000 new cancer cases are diagnosed each year, and 547,000 people die of cancer. People who outlive their cancers can only be diagnosed retrospectively, when they die years later from another cause.

A true survivor measures life by its quality, rather than by its length. People who spend years brooding on their disease, and waiting for it to recur, may die of something else in the end: however, they are never truly cured.

YOUR CONTINUING RELATIONSHIP WITH THE HOSPITAL

Shocking though the cancer diagnosis has been, it is usually delivered in the womb-like security of the hospital. It is followed by a period of intensive treatment, when the medical staff and your friends and family will focus a lot of love, care and attention on you. But then the day comes when you have recovered from your operation and/or your courses of radiotherapy and chemotherapy. You are discharged as 'well' and told you can resume normal life, although you will need to return for periodic check-ups.

Your friends and family will be delighted that the worst is over. From now on the whole world seems to be expecting you to get on with the business of your recovery. But far from 'getting on with it', it may be only now that you have the time and space to consider what has happened to you.

Sharon, 47, was determined to remain cool and in control throughout her treatment for invasive cervical cancer. She explained: 'I had opened the letter from my family doctor to the consultant and already knew my diagnosis. I asked the specialist to be totally straight with me and told him I could take it. I was a model patient all the time I was in hospital, and the doctors, nurses, friends and family all said how well I was doing.'

When Sharon was told she would not need another check-up for three months, she felt full of confidence and embarked on an ambitious keep-fit programme. Several weeks later she noticed a swelling in her groin and a pain in her hip. However, she was told it would be a month before she could see the consultant again.

'I was convinced the lump was the cancer eating away at me, and I flew into a complete panic. I insisted on hand delivering a note on to the consultant's desk which said that if he couldn't see me *immediately*, he must arrange radiotherapy as the cancer had come back.'

The consultant saw Sharon that week and reassured her the swelling and pain were side effects of all the vigorous physical exercises she had been doing.

Cancer specialists say such false alarms are common. Nevertheless, expecting urgent attention for an unexpected symptom is not a sign of panic, but a sensible precaution.

Most people who are treated for cancer continue to be followed up by the hospital, often for life. At first you are likely to have monthly appointments, but as you progress the intervals will get longer. These check-ups will often include tests to see if the cancer has come back, and waiting for the results will inevitably cause anxiety.

But even if all your check-ups are clear, you may suddenly start to worry about a recurrence, years after a successful treatment. If this happens, you may find it difficult to confide in anyone when the whole world thinks you are mentally and physically recovered from your cancer. This surfacing of worry is not your body telling you something is wrong, but a sign that your suppressed anxieties have floated to the surface.

Psychiatrists advise that whenever we have a particular worry, we do everything we can to alleviate it and then shut the door on it. This is obviously easier to say than to do, but some strategies for dealing with your natural fear of recurrence are described in Chapter 8 (see page 93). One of the most upsetting aspects of a cancer diagnosis is the loss of personal control it represents. When you go back for a check-up, you inevitably have to sit around waiting to be seen, or to hear the results of tests. Once again, you can feel you have lost control of your future.

This is distressing and it is not surprising that many people forget their carefully prepared questions once they see the doctor or nurse.

Remember the consultation is for your benefit – and try to work out in advance what you want to get out of it. Although your family doctor can help you at any time, it is the hospital doctor who will be able to answer your questions with most authority, and order any necessary checks most quickly.

In the weeks preceding your check-up, note down any unexpected symptoms or questions you want to ask, and keep the list with your hospital appointment card so it is not forgotten. Even if you don't need the list, because the doctor or nurse volunteers the information, preparing the questions helps you regain some control.

The delayed effects of radiotherapy and chemotherapy treatments can easily be mistaken for a recurrence of your cancer, unless you are warned about them. For example, it is quite common for radiotherapy to lead to persistent diarrhoea, or a dry cough, many weeks after the treatment has finished. More details about the after-effects of treatment are given in Chapter 6 (see page 61).

Although you should be warned about these symptoms, this does not always happen. It is wise to double-check if there are likely to be any delayed effects. Make sure you ask how common these effects are, too. They may only affect a minority of people. Also, ask if there are any specific symptoms you should watch out for as an early warning that your cancer has returned.

The most important question for every cancer patient is 'Will I get better?' If your treatment has been palliative (to reduce your symptoms rather than attempt to remove the cancer), you will want to know, 'How long have I got?' You may have held back from asking these questions during your hospital treatment, but will now feel an overwhelming desire for some answers.

It is a good rule in life never to ask a question, unless you are sure you want to know the answer. But often we *are* sure. We need to make plans, reassign priorities and sort out our affairs. If you really want to know, don't hesitate to ask. Often, the truth is less frightening that whatever you are imagining.

Don't be surprised, however, if the reply is hedged. Doctors are constantly being surprised by their patients. People who are given a gloomy prognosis often make it a point of pride to prove the consultant wrong. The course of some cancers is much easier to predict than others, and new, relatively untried treatments can also complicate the situation. Nevertheless, it should be possible to get an idea about whether your future is likely to be measured in weeks, months or years. Doctors and patients often view cancer in a very different way: for a doctor a treatment that increases a patient's chances of survival by ten per cent is well worth trying.

John, 50, who was given chemotherapy to treat his bowel cancer, asked his consultant how much difference it would make to his chances of survival. 'I suppose I expected him to say 90 per cent,' said John. 'Actually it was 17 per cent, which disappointed me – although the doctor seemed to think that was really good.'

If your treatment has been completed, you may feel dismayed that your doctor appears to have lost interest in you. You can psych yourself up for a follow-up visit, only to find that you see a different doctor who may seem insensitive or simply uninterested. If you are further along the road to recovery, you may actually miss the regular, intense check-ups. Although they were a nuisance at the time, they did mean that something was being done about your cancer.

Debbie, diagnosed with breast cancer at 43, said: 'One of the worst things about having cancer was the feeling that I had lost the sense of ownership of my body. I had become a set of symptoms associated with a defective breast. Yet when my nine months of treatment came to an end, I felt as if I had been cast adrift.'

According to the Cancer Research Campaign, patients frequently complain that when they do return for a check-up, doctors are in too much of a hurry to tell them everything they need to know. It can be very difficult for medical staff to gauge exactly the right amount of information to give. If they tell you every side effect of radiotherapy, they may cause unnecessary alarm. Indeed, you may be so scared that you want to abandon a treatment that could save your life.

An even greater problem is the fact that individuals vary a great deal in how much they want to know. Some people prefer to leave the details to the doctors, while others strive to acquire a very detailed knowledge of their condition and treatment options.

Anger towards the hospital or the staff is a common reaction. Sometimes it is well justified, and sometimes it is really an expression of rage over what has happened. Suzanne was angry with the way her consultant had told her that her cancer of the pancreas was impossible to treat. She said: 'He could have said that although things didn't look good, some patients do better than others, and that he was often surprised. Instead, he left me with no hope.'

Suzanne, who was 52, also had another bone to pick with the specialist. The leaflet he had given her about painkillers had said she would not become addicted to the morphine she needed to control her pain. One day, she forgot to take her tablets, and suffered agitation and terrors as a result of drug withdrawal. 'Why do they pretend morphine is not addictive, when it is?' she asked.

The problem is the same one that John encountered when he enquired about how much difference chemotherapy would make: doctors and patients do not always speak the same language. There is no doubt that anyone who takes large doses of morphine over a long period risks becoming physically dependent on it and will need to be weaned off slowly. To a doctor, the medical definition of addiction is that someone becomes psychologically dependent on the drug – and this is not what happens with cancer patients. When people no longer need heroin, the doses are gradually reduced over a period of time, and physical dependence does not occur either.

The leaflet was not intended to con Suzanne and other patients, but her anger had led her to lose her sense of perspective. Suggesting to the consultant that patients need to be given some hope during a diagnosis, and asking for a better explanation in the leaflet would have been less destructive to Suzanne than her simmering anger. More information about dealing with anger is given in Chapter 8 (see page 93).

GETTING INFORMATION

You have a right to information about your condition. It is in the doctor's interests to provide this, because if you understand what is going on, you are more likely to co-operate with the treatment. If he or she is not telling you what you need to know, then it is a good idea to make this clear (tactfully) to the consultant, or one of the more sympathetic members of the medical staff. Many hospitals now provide booklets or other written material to explain your treatment. If yours does not, it is worth asking why.

Cancer support organizations such as BACUP (the British Association of Cancer-United Patients) and the American Cancer Society (see Useful Addresses, page 147) provide detailed information about different types of cancer, and what you can expect from various treatments.

If you read medical textbooks in the public library, check when they were published (this information is usually given on the copyright page of the book). Cancer treatments have advanced a great deal in the last decade, and an outdated textbook could cause you a lot of unnecessary grief and alarm. Even if your textbook is up to date, be prepared for the fact that the prognosis may make gloomy reading. This, along with any survival statistics given, is a generalization, and does not necessarily apply to your particular case.

QUESTIONS FOR YOUR DOCTOR

- Can I expect any delayed effects of treatment?
- What are the warning signs that my cancer is recurring?
- What is the likely outcome of my treatment?
- How can I get more information about my condition?

People with cancer are often bombarded with information about different alternative treatments, special diets and herbal remedies – and so are their nearest and dearest. This information overload can lead you to latch on to any therapist, book or article that offers a definite opinion.

Linda, a 45-year-old breast cancer patient, decided to reject the radiotherapy and chemotherapy that her doctor had recommended after reading an article in an alternative health magazine. The magazine had been quite categorical in stating that these additional treatments made no difference to the patient's expected life span. 'The article was absolutely definite and no one else was,' she said.

Who could blame Linda for latching on to a simple statement when her doctors could not offer a black and white guarantee that further treatment would help her live longer? Unfortunately, the article was not truly authoritative, but simply prejudiced against mainstream medicine.

DEPRESSION AS A STAGING POINT

Psychiatrists say we go through the same kinds of stages after a cancer diagnosis as when we are bereaved. First we experience shock (which may be expressed as bitter distress, numbness or by not appearing to react at all); then there is depression (which may be expressed in the form of fear and anger as well as sadness); and finally there is acceptance of the situation, and a desire to move on.

You may not fit exactly into this pattern, but most people with cancer will experience periods of pessimism and depression. More information about this is given in Chapter 2 (see page 20).

Dr Rosy Daniels, a qualified doctor and a holistic medical practitioner at Bristol Cancer Help Centre, believes the medical profession is partly to blame for making cancer patients depressed. She explains: 'Doctors tend to treat cancer as an inexorable process, as if nothing you can do will make any difference. It is a big message and you need to wipe it out of your psyche. You have a physical repair system which needs to be rediscovered, because the nurturing and self-healing part of medicine has been left out of the picture.'

Dr Daniels adds that when you emerge from your personal Slough of Despond, cancer can galvanize you into action. 'It can be a gift in disguise, although a very painful gift which none of us would have chosen.'

CHAPTER 2

GETTING BACK TO NORMAL

But all went well! The operation proved
First possible, and then a great success!
Reprieve – for years of shameless diaries
I had resolved to burn. Oxfam must
wait for all those clothes.

(SHARON WILLMOTT, AFTER HER OPERATION FOR
CERVICAL CANCER)

LIFE AFTER TREATMENT

Once your treatment is over, your friends and family are likely to breathe a sigh of relief. 'At last you can get back to normal,' they will say. But the fact is that for many people with cancer, life will never be normal again. This is not to say it will not be joyous, or exciting, or unpredictable. But it is unlikely to be quite the same.

Your ability to cope, so useful at the time of diagnosis, can now become a real burden. If everyone is praising you 'for managing so well' and telling you 'I could never have been so brave' it is difficult to admit that, weeks or months after the treatment, you are neither managing nor feeling brave. Working through some very negative and painful feelings, or simply taking stock, can be difficult when the rest of the world thinks the book has been closed.

Some people cope by taking an obsessive interest in the latest cancer research. For them, the false dawns offered by stories of 'breakthroughs' can be crushing. A handful of cancers can already be cured, and more progress is being made, mainly in the fine tuning of treatments. But our understanding of the causes and prevention of cancer still lies in the future. Most people reading this book are more likely to benefit from the results of the latest psychological research than from the scientists' quest for the 'magic' compound.

THE POWER OF POSITIVE THINKING

Many mainstream doctors are now accepting that no matter how brilliant the surgery and drug treatments, their patients will never be truly healthy if they are psychologically distressed. But what is the best way of overcoming the negative feelings that can so easily undermine the healing process?

Dr Stephen Greer, one of the most distinguished researchers into the links between mental attitude and cancer notes that even when the physical symptoms of cancer disappear, many patients suffer extreme depression and anxiety caused by fears of recurrence. Dr Greer, a consultant psychiatrist at the Royal Marsden Hospital, London, was one of the first mainstream doctors to show that a fighting spirit or simple denial increases a patient's chances of survival.

His more recent research has shown that therapies that reduce feelings of helplessness, focus on a patient's individual strengths, induce a fighting spirit and help to promote feelings of personal control improve psychological health. This work has not continued long enough to show an increase in longevity. However, the quality of life is undoubtedly improved by this type of psychological support.

COGNITIVE THERAPY

The objective of cognitive therapy is to turn negative thoughts into positive ones that will aid your recovery. Self-help treatments which encourage people to be less passive have been shown to help them cope better with the disease, and suffer less distress. Whether such treatments can help you to live longer as well remains highly controversial and is discussed in Chapter 8 (see page 93). However, for many people, feeling happier and more in control of their lives may be enough.

Facing up to cancer is particularly difficult and painful for people who blame themselves for everything that goes wrong in their lives. This type of negative-self talk, where people accuse themselves of being stupid, incompetent or generally worthless, is fairly common. This critical inner voice undermines our self-worth, and can make us feel helpless and hopeless – a dangerous frame of mind for a cancer patient.

Cognitive therapy teaches you to challenge the false beliefs and negative thoughts that are making you unhappy and delaying your recovery. You may find that you are naturally practising some of these techniques anyway – even if you have never heard of them.

Renée, 66, had no idea what visualization was, and said she had not tried any complementary therapies. She recounted: 'It sounds silly, but every night, I lie in bed and imagine that any rotten cells which may be in my body are leaving by my feet – and they're not coming back.' In fact, Renée, who was treated for facial cancer, is practising a form of visualization, in which the imagination is harnessed in the fight against disease.

Further conversation revealed that Renée also practises positive thinking and cognitive therapy as well: 'The surgeon had to take my nose away, and I now have a prosthesis. I don't worry about the disfigurement – if people look at me, then let them look. I don't think they realize the nose is false, but my face is a little swollen at the sides, as if I've been in an accident.

'When I remove my prosthesis, I don't think about cancer – cleaning it is just another little chore, like cleaning your teeth. I believe very strongly that if you allow yourself to think negative thoughts, you can wish the cancer back on yourself. I get apprehensive before check-ups and those are the times when I just have to talk very sternly to myself, remind myself that I am feeling well, and that the surgeon says he thinks he got all the cancer when he operated.'

Some people cope with cancer by denying they have the disease, or by minimizing it – explaining they are only having a mastectomy, for instance, 'in case there is a malignancy'. Denial of the seriousness of the situation may be a good survival approach, although this is seldom publicized because it fits less neatly into the various theories about how cancer patients should think or behave. Denial is one way of regaining control in what seems to be an impossible situation, and it protects you against thinking that every minor symptom is a recurrence of your disease. But neither complementary nor conventional therapists recommend it as a survival strategy.

When Jim, 68, was told his cancer of the oesophagus was

inoperable, he flatly denied it, telling the doctor: 'That's just your opinion and not mine.' Afterwards, Jim explained: 'I would be lying if I said I was not concerned by what the doctor told me and I did immediately check my wife would be able to get my retirement pension. But I am not frightened because I am 100 per cent convinced I can beat this. I have accepted defeat in no other aspect of my life, and this is just another challenge which I have to meet. I think the main cure for cancer lies within yourself. The mind is very powerful. You can convince yourself of something and make it happen for good or bad. I am making long-term plans – planting bulbs to come up next spring.'

Jim is not relying solely on his own resources, however. He has had radiotherapy to relieve his symptoms, attends regular check-ups, and plans to have chemotherapy if necessary.

Both Renée and Jim have worked out their own forms of cognitive therapy, but their reaction is unusual. Many cancer patients would benefit from techniques that help them deal with their diagnosis and communicate more easily with their friends and family.

Cognitive therapy can be particularly helpful in dealing with problems such as a change in body shape, function or appearance, sexual problems, intense anger or anticipatory nausea and vomiting (experienced by some people who have had chemotherapy, whenever they approach their hospital).

When cognitive therapy is given as part of structured psychotherapy treatment, it involves up to 12 weekly sessions of an hour. You may be treated by a psychiatrist, a psychologist or another trained health professional.

During this time you will have the opportunity to: express your feelings to someone who encourages you to talk, and does not tell you what you should be thinking; learn to structure your day; deal with false beliefs; and challenge negative thoughts.

Some large cancer centres offer cognitive therapy, and many more offer psychological support. If you feel you need this type of help, you should ring the unit where your cancer has been treated. In the UK, the cancer charity BACUP can provide free counselling in its London and Edinburgh offices, and also advise you on how to find a therapist. In the US, the American Cancer Society can provide similar help. Another US agency, Cancer Care, provides a free counselling service. For contact numbers see Useful Addresses, page 147.

SELF-HELP COGNITIVE THERAPY

If you are unable to find a therapist, or you simply do not wish to, then you can devise your own treatment. To do this you will need to work through several stages.

STEPS IN SELF-HELP COGNITIVE THERAPY

- Ventilate your feelings
- Regain control of your life
- Deal with false beliefs
- Avoid negative thinking
- Make sense of your experience

The first stage is to decide how to ventilate your feelings. Many people find complementary therapists are helpful listeners. Others go to support groups where cancer patients can provide mutual comfort, encouragement and understanding. Although close friends, partners and family members can be helpful they can sometimes be too close. This may make it difficult for you to air your feelings in case you alarm them. Sometimes those close to you feel, wrongly, that it is better to change the subject. Sometimes they find your cancer too painful to discuss.

If you feel you have lost control over your life, you need to schedule in some activities or challenges to structure your day. Make a list of the hobbies and pleasures you have given up since you were diagnosed, and decide which ones you want to reinstate. Make a general wish list.

If one day drags into another, and you find yourself getting into a vicious circle where you get up later and do less and less each day, you can regain control and a sense of achievement by making a daily activity plan. The activities can be very simple, such as cleaning the car, sorting out a cupboard, starting an evening class, seeing a therapist, finishing an abandoned project, getting up early to be first in the queue for the sales, learning to use a new computer program, decorating a room. Everyone's wish list will be different. If all of these sound dire, think of something which suits you better!

Don't blame yourself if you don't get through the list. The point of the exercise is to reinstate some objectives, not to drive yourself into the ground. Most importantly, make sure you schedule in some enjoyment as well. If you are too low to contemplate following this advice, see the section on depression (page 29).

Another important strategy is to deal with false beliefs by challenging the thoughts and fears that worry you most. For instance, if you think your wife finds you less attractive because of your orchiectomy (or your husband is put off by your mastectomy), then ask your partner what she or he really thinks. The very worst thing that can happen is that your fears will be justified. However, it is much more likely that they are unfounded, even though your partner may initially have been badly shocked by what has happened to you. Indeed, your partner may have been looking for a way of reassuring you on this point, but did not know the right words to use. More information about cancer and sexual relationships is given in Chapter 5 (see page 50).

If you have convinced yourself your doctor is lying to you, then test this belief by speaking to the doctor again, or double-checking with another doctor. Whatever the answer, it will not be worse than your fears.

We often use false beliefs against ourselves, thinking in terms of 'shoulds' and 'musts'. For instance, you may tell yourself that you *should* not be a burden on others, or that you *must* get through your therapy without making a fuss. When you find yourself using absolute words such as should, must, always, incredibly, totally, never and always, then try exchanging them for could, might, sometimes, quite, very, seldom and often. Then ask yourself if even this expression is going too far.

One way of challenging such views is to ask yourself whether you would expect such standards of others. Would you feel that a friend had no right to burden you with his or her worries during an illness, or that a relative must never complain about an unpleasant treatment?

Negative thinking can creep up on the most positive of people, particularly when they are feeling low. If you are the type of person who expects to look after other people, rather than be cared for, then your self-image may be so damaged by the cancer diagnosis that you are at particular risk.

Dwelling on negative thoughts is like shooting yourself in the foot. We become persuaded our lives have run out of control and there is nothing we can do to take charge of our own destiny. But in fact, nearly every negative thought can be examined, and turned into a more positive reaction. Once again, if you consider your situation as if it involved another person, you are likely to take a more realistic view. Write down some negative thoughts, and then consider how you might turn them round. For example,

> *I am in a truly terrible situation*
> can be turned into
> *Things are never quite as bad as they seem at first.*

> *I always mess things up, and now I've arrived at the hospital*
> *on the wrong day*
> becomes
> *I make mistakes sometimes, but so do other people –*
> *particularly when they are upset, as I am.*

> *I'm a coward about death – I can't change the way I am*
> is turned into
> *If I choose, I can change the way I view life and death, and I*
> *can change the way I react to stressful situations.*

Many doctors say the patients who cope best put their illness on the 'back burner', return to normal life, and only occasionally think about their cancers. Some people do this more easily than others, and research is currently under way to identify how this is achieved, so that others can follow suit. However, Dr Amanda Ramirez, consultant psychiatrist at Guy's Hospital, London, emphasizes that simply trying to shut out the cancer is unlikely to be effective.

One of the most important aspects of self-help cognitive therapy is making sense of what has happened to you. Dr Ramirez explains: 'People may come through their treatment looking neither to the left nor the right, but they will then need to make sense of the wider issues. Their values may well have changed, and they may have new priorities. Cancer can expose the weaknesses and strengths in a relationship. Before you can put your cancer on the back burner, you have to try and make some sense of what has happened, and accept the possibility that the disease may come back. It's a question of sorting it out first, and then putting it away.'

AVOIDING POISONOUS PEOPLE

But it isn't only the critical, nagging inner voice that can delay your recovery. Some people are almost literally poisonous – and if anyone has a right to avoid them at this vulnerable time in your life, then you do. You don't need to hear a series of anecdotes about people who died of cancer 20 years ago, having suffered horribly!

Others are poisonous by accident. Relatives for whom cancer is the Disease which Dare not Speak its Name, and who talk about your 'little operation', can sap your energy. There is no need for you to play this game, or join the conspiracy of silence. And you also need to be prepared for occasions when people open their mouths without first engaging the brain.

Sally, 55, was telling a friend how good she felt about getting the all-clear after her five-year check-up.'It was a real watershed for me, but my friend said, "That's good, but it's not five years – it's seven." I thought about that, and felt really depressed. Then I reminded myself that the people who really know about my disease, the doctors, had said that being clear for five years was a very good sign indeed. I think it's important to be prepared for what people might say to you, because otherwise you can be knocked back so easily.' More information about dealing with other people is given in Chapter 3 (see page 33).

EMOTIONALLY VULNERABLE PEOPLE

Some people are naturally at higher risk of psychological problems when they are diagnosed with cancer. For example, people who do not have a close, confiding relationship with another person may find it difficult to talk about their true feelings – or to get their problems into perspective. Likewise, people who were deprived love as children may find it difficult to adjust to life once they are discharged from hospital.

Dr Amanda Ramirez explains: 'For people who have had bad childhoods, hospital may provide their first experience of being cared for and nurtured. Every day, a doctor or nurse will ask how they are, and will minister to their needs. If they found it difficult to make friends normally, they will have enjoyed the camaraderie of a ward where, however difficult and unpleasant the treatments, everyone is going through the same thing. They may feel bereft of this love and support when they are back out in the world again.'

If you are already dealing with another life crisis such as a shaky marriage, homelessness, or the loss of a parent, you may try to shelve your cancer before you have had time to come to terms with it. Some chemotherapy drugs can leave you emotionally as well as physically fragile. Younger patients generally seem to be more susceptible to psychological illness than older people.

Finally, if you spend your professional or personal life absorbed in caring for other people, you may find it hard to allow yourself to be a person who requires care. Jean's story illustrates this perfectly. She was an occupational health nurse. Like many people whose work involves caring for others, she found it difficult to give herself permission to be ill, or to find the time and space she needed for her cancer.

She returned to work in the two weeks between her cancer diagnosis and her mastectomy because she wanted to show a positive example to the women in her factory. 'I wanted them to realize that that breast cancer didn't make you disappear.'

Five weeks after her mastectomy she returned to work. 'I thought I was over it, and then the depression hit me like a brick wall.' After a year on antidepressants – during which Jean has practised stress reduction and relaxation techniques – she said: 'I'm still in the early stages of recovery, but I'm working on it.'

Dr Rosy Daniels commented: 'Some people believe they have recovered from their cancer as soon as they are physically fit again. They then want to go and organize the Women's Institute or run a support group and look after lots of other people. They are filled with the desire to help others, but they are not really ready for that, because they have not dealt with their cancer, and they have not given themselves a chance to heal.'

Some people have no real incentive to get well, because they believe their illness is the most interesting thing about them, or because they enjoy the safety and security that the hospital provides.

Jamie had been put in care at seven, after his mother walked out and his father proved unable to cope with him. He had been unable to settle down with foster parents, and spent most of his remaining childhood in care. At the age of 22 he developed leukaemia, and spent 14 months almost permanently in hospital.

But far from experiencing a sense of release on discharge from hospital, Jamie became unhappy and unsettled at home in his flat. He constantly returned to the ward, to visit other patients and talk to the medical and nursing staff. He attended the funerals of anyone who had been on the ward. Only life on the ward, and the activities of patients and nursing staff, counted as real life to him.

He explained to his psychiatrist that his job as a messenger seemed meaningless, and he could not understand why people got so worked up about things he knew to be trivial. When people complained, he wanted to shake them by the neck and shout: 'You're fit and healthy, and you'll be alive next year. How dare you complain all the time.'

The nursing staff on his ward were becoming unhappy about the emotional demands Jamie was making on them, and were now discouraging his visits. Jamie was distraught. His psychiatrist offered to help, but warned that the therapy to try to break Jamie of his dependency would involve exploring painful events from his past. Jamie had already lost his job, and alienated his friends, and decided he had nothing to lose by going ahead with the therapy.

DEALING WITH DEPRESSION

Nearly everyone needs time to adjust to having cancer, but for about one person in four this adjustment can be particularly painful, and the individuals concerned suffer from clinically significant anxiety and depression. It may be that some people do not give themselves time to adjust to the changes which cancer brings to their lives. More than 50 per cent of women who have a mastectomy return to work within three months of their operations.

In the previous section, we described how cancer can be a time for change and growth. But these positive changes can only occur when the depression is left behind. Sinking into the doldrums for a while is natural. But if your depression lingers, no amount of well-meaning advice to 'pull yourself together' will help. If you could have done it by yourself, you would have done so.

Many people are reluctant to seek help because they are afraid of seeming weak in the eyes of the world. But none of us would condemn a friend who needed medical help for cancer-induced depression, so why are we so hard on ourselves?

As Dr Rosy Daniels points out, if you sink below a certain point you are simply unable to help yourself: 'You can go into a negative spiral where you feel depressed and so anxious that your pain levels rise, and any symptoms seem much worse. In that phase, you need a tremendous amount of input before you are strong enough to help yourself.'

Dr Daniels counsels against wasting energy by keeping up a falsely brave face. 'We British are bad about accepting our vulnerability, and too embarrassed to ask for help, and yet if we break a leg, we accept people running around for us. You can lose valuable energy keeping things looking as if they are OK when they are not.'

She believes that complementary therapies such as visualization and relaxation play a vital role in recovery from cancer. However, trying to practise them alone at home, when your morale is at rock bottom, she warns, is doomed to failure.

'Complementary therapies work by unblocking the energy so you can re-integrate your body, mind and spirit. You will need a lot of input from others – healers and therapists – and you may need to practise some of your therapies in a class with others rather than trying to manage at home. One day you will wake up, knowing you can take on these processes for yourself. You could end up beating yourself up because you haven't got the energy or motivation to go through with it. You need the help of therapists, and you really need to be in a class with others.'

Dr Maurice Slevin works in a centre where counselling, psychotherapy, relaxation and massage are offered as complementary therapies. Although he believes patients find them helpful, there are times, he says, when antidepressant drugs play an important role.

He explains: 'People wonder why it is necessary to consider antidepressants. After all, depression in the face of cancer is a natural reaction, and the antidepressants cannot change the course of the disease. I would agree that feeling low for a while does not warrant treatment. But if depression really sets in, people can sink so far that they are unable to cope with everyday life. This can blight the recovery of someone whose cancer is curable, or in lengthy remission. Once people are no longer regularly coming to the hospital for check-ups or treatment, they have to face up to their anxieties. Often, they feel they should be happy and end up feeling upset.

'In most people these feelings last only for a short time, and acknowledging them, and realizing such feelings are normal, all help them to move to the next phase. But when these feelings linger, I think antidepressants are needed. As a guideline, if you are feeling a bit miserable, thinking negatively but getting on with your life, then you may not need drug treatment – unless these feelings linger for two or three months. However, if depression is so severe that you are crying all the time and can't be bothered to get up and dressed in the morning, then you need help quickly. If things are really bad, a friend or relative may need to call a doctor out to see you. Depression is an illness and should be treated as such.'

If five of the items listed below apply to you – including depressed mood or a loss of interest or pleasure – then you should see your family doctor. If you keep thinking of suicide, you must get help regardless of how you score with other items on the list.

1 Depressed mood
2 Marked loss of interest or pleasure in daily activities
3 Feelings of worthlessness or excessive and inappropriate guilt
4 Significant weight loss or gain that cannot be explained by dieting, your cancer or your treatment
5 Insomnia, early waking in the morning or, conversely, excessive desire to sleep
6 Fatigue or loss of energy that cannot be explained by your condition or treatment
7 Reduced ability to think clearly or concentrate
8 Early morning miseries and mood swings during the day
9 Jerky limb movements, or very slow movements
10 Frequent thoughts of suicide

If you do need antidepressants, they work best if you take a full dose for at least six weeks. Your doctor will then probably reduce the dose and want you to continue for four to six months. Many people want to stop earlier than this, but research has shown that the treatment works much better – and recurrence of depression is less likely – with longer courses of drugs. It may take several weeks before you feel the benefits of antidepressants and they can produce unpleasant side effects such as stomach upsets, dry mouth and lassitude. If this happens, the dose should be reduced or the drug changed.

Antidepressants are in a different class of drugs from tranquillizers, and you are extremely unlikely to become dependent on them. However, if you are unable to function normally because of disabling anxiety, you may need to take tranquillizers despite the risk of dependency. In these circumstances, tranquillizers are most useful before and during an anxiety-provoking situation (such as chemotherapy) rather than on a daily basis. Some people find that relaxation techniques (see page 117) work just as well for them as drugs. More information on how you can use your mental attitude to fight cancer is given in Chapter 8 (see page 93).

CHAPTER 3

DEALING WITH OTHER PEOPLE

*Of course, everyone who has cancer would much prefer
not to have it, or to be cured of it . . . the contact between
you and your friends can be an extraordinary and
wonderful proof of the value of human companionship.
Serious illness may threaten a life, but it does not rob that
life of meaning.*

DR ROBERT BUCKMAN AND JOHN ELSEGOOD, WHO CAN EVER
UNDERSTAND? BACUP BOOKLET

YOUR NEAREST AND DEAREST

You may feel you have enough to worry about, without having to
think about the feelings and reactions of those closest to you. Yet
you *need* them. Research has shown that people with no one to
confide in are more likely to suffer anxiety and depression –
negative emotions that delay their recovery. If we have pent-up
feelings like anger or sadness, it becomes difficult to talk about
anything normally until those feelings are acknowledged and
expressed.

Most of us have a natural instinct not to impose our feelings
on others. Perhaps you are wondering if it is unfair to confide in
your nearest and dearest at all. After all they have just come
through the trauma of your diagnosis and first wave of treatment.
Might it not be better better to soldier on alone now the first
flurry of excitement over your cancer has passed?

For a small minority of people, this will be the right choice.
These people enjoy their self-sufficiency and thrive on their own
counsel. But if you are solitary by circumstance rather than by
choice, you do not need to carry on alone. There are plenty of

support groups around that will welcome you as a member and value your input.

SUPPORT GROUPS

Many people who are surrounded by caring friends and relatives also find it a relief to share their feelings and experiences with a support group. People who have been through similar experiences are less likely to be embarrassed by your grief and anger, or to want to try and stop you from airing a painful experience.

Sometimes the cancer unit responsible for your treatment will run its own support group (although you are not obliged to join it), or will know of something suitable locally. Telephone counselling, and some face to face counselling, is also arranged by the British charity BACUP. The BACUP counsellors, or the charity CancerLink, may also be able to put you in touch with a local support group, or you may find one immediately by simply checking your phone book under Cancer.

In the US you can find a local support group by calling the social-work department of your hospital or a national resource centre such as the National Cancer Institute, American Cancer Society, or the National Coalition for Cancer Survivorship. Your local newspaper may publish a list of support groups in your area. For names and numbers, see Useful Addresses (page 147).

People with cancer often say that no one can really understand their feelings as well as someone else who has gone through the same experience. Kathleen Sheridan Russell, who runs support groups for BACUP, says: 'The people in the greatest need of a group are often the ones whose treatment has finished. They can feel very much on their own, especially as everyone wants them to be over their cancer. Their friends and family are telling them they look great and that makes it hard for them to admit that they are really feeling weepy and vulnerable. That's where a support group comes into its own.

'In our groups we give people the space to really go into why, for instance, they are afraid of dying. Many people realize their family would get distressed if they tried to discuss it with them. The support group gives them the chance to discuss their fears, and discover that others feel exactly the same. That helps to normalize their feelings.

'People with cancer get irritated when well-meaning friends

comment that none of us know how long we've got to liv
they could be run over by a bus tomorrow. How man
really get run over by buses? The cancer patient is grappl
a genuine and justified worry about survival, which other cancer
patients in the group can understand.'

Support groups are not for everyone, and one may suit you
much better than another, so you may need to try several. Be
suspicious of any organization that claims to cure cancer, or is
offering a high-priced product, or that actively encourages you to
abandon conventional treatment (there is a world of difference
between a group which supports any decision you make, and one
which tries to make up your mind for you).

Remember that because of the uncertainties of cancer, you
and those close to you make easy victims for the plausible
charlatan. Whatever the prognosis of your cancer, its very
existence is likely to make you think about death. Yet this is one
of the last twentieth-century taboos, and one which your family
may find particularly difficult to discuss with you.

DIFFICULTIES IN CONFIDING

For many of us, our family and friends will play an important role
in the recovery process. However, talking to them can be difficult.
Perhaps you do not belong to the 'caring, sharing' generation that
discusses feelings freely. Cancer does not mean you have to
abandon your privacy, but if you do feel you want to talk to
someone, you may find it difficult to know where to begin.

You may be afraid that if you talk to people about how you
really feel, they will be disappointed at your lack of stoicism, or
embarrassed because they don't know what to say. There is no
denying that social taboos still surround any discussion of a life-
threatening illness – although these barriers are slowly being
broken down.

You may fear that you will burst into tears. You may even have
the superstitious belief that if you do discuss the future, or talk
about the possibility of recurrence, you will somehow make it
happen. Unless your nearest and dearest are exceptionally tactful
and sensitive people, they may find it difficult to strike the right
note. Because of this they will feel clumsy and uncertain, and may
become easily offended if you appear to reject their efforts.

Sharon, 46, had just returned home after receiving treatment for cervical cancer when her brother-in-law phoned.

'He was obviously embarrassed that I had answered the phone. He said, "Sharon, I've heard about your little trouble." He just didn't know what to say. I replied, "Yes, it's a bugger, isn't it," and you could hear the sigh of relief down the phone, that I was still talking in the same way, and still using the same bad language.'

CANCER FROM THE OTHER SIDE

Your cancer diagnosis and treatment was a personal crisis: it is easy to overlook the shock and disorientation experienced by your nearest and dearest. However, now that the immediate crisis is over, it is useful to consider the cancer experience from your family's point of view. This understanding will give you a better chance of helping them to help you.

Your family and friends will have experienced many of the things you have experienced – disbelief, bewilderment, anger, denial, grief, insomnia, depression, anxiety and, worst of all, a loss of control of their lives. You have changed, in their eyes, from a strong and healthy person to a vulnerable one with an uncertain future. And because they have not had cancer themselves, they may have felt forced to bottle up their feelings rather than risk making you feel worse than you do already.

Loved ones may protect themselves by going into a type of premature mourning. Your partner may become angry at the prospect of having to manage without you, even though he or she knows such anger is irrational. You may need to pick up on this and say that you are not ready to leave this world yet, and you want them to support you, rather than write you off.

Sharon found that six months after her successful treatment, her husband had become rather distant: 'I realized he had expected me to die, which wasn't surprising, because my surgeon had been pessimistic and I had certainly thought I was going to die. My husband had made contingency plans, and started to think about what was going to happen after I had gone. Now he had realized he was going to have to readjust to the idea that I was around after all.'

INTIMATIONS OF MORTALITY

Your diagnosis has not only forced your nearest and dearest to consider what life might be like without you, but also to confront the unthinkable – their own mortality. In the long run, this can have positive effects on family relationships as people realize how important it is to value the time they have together, and to avoid meaningless petty squabbles.

However, most people who are close to a cancer patient will experience some 'survivor guilt'. You may ask, 'Why me?' but they will equally ask, 'Why not me?' Some of the tears they shed will be for themselves and the impact of your cancer on their lives. This can lead to feelings of shame that they are thinking of themselves when they feel they should be thinking about you. Such mixed feelings can lead to bitter arguments between family members who accuse each other of not supporting you properly. They cannot handle their grief and uncertainty about the future, so they are resorting to the 'easier' emotions of anger and disgust with each other.

Far from being helped, you may find yourself in the role of bridge-builder and peacemaker, acknowledging that these have been difficult times and asking them to reconsider for your sake. In extreme cases, you may conclude the game is not worth the candle and chop them out of your lives. It is up to you to decide which option is most likely to assist your recovery. Some friends and family members will fall by the wayside, overwhelmed by their own fear of cancer. Try not to take it too personally if they avoid you: cancer phobia is their problem not yours and their own limitations make it impossible for them to be any use to you at this time.

'LET'S FORGET ALL ABOUT IT'

It is likely that now your treatment is over your nearest and dearest will (consciously or unconsciously) want to forget all about your cancer. They would love to pretend it never happened (as you probably would too). At the same time they will be living with the same uncertainty that nearly all cancer patients experience about whether the disease will come back.

Sometimes the partner of a cancer patient will refuse to accept the seriousness of the situation. This can be frustrating and infuriating, and prevent you from expresssing your fears on days when you are feeling low. Dr Amanda Ramirez explained: 'One of the most difficult counselling situations occurs when the patient's partner is wildly optimistic about the future, while the patient has a more realistic view. It is often caused because the partner cannot face up to the possibility that the loved one will die. As therapists, we cannot baldly put this to the partner. The skill of the psychotherapist lies in helping the partner understand why he or she feels the way he or she does.'

RECURRENCE

If your disease recurs at some later stage, some of your closest friends and family may feel guilty that they didn't persuade you to follow a particular course of treatment or diet. They may feel anger towards the medical experts for failing to provide a cure – and they may be inclined to write you off.

Your friends and family are likely to be devastated by a recurrence of your disease, and possibly treat it as a death sentence rather than a setback. Some of them may try to distance themselves (premature mourning again) by talking to your doctors and nurses rather than to you. Once again, you may need to remind them not to write you off. Some survivors and their families experience a series of recurrences of their disease – with each one being controlled by surgery, chemotherapy or radiotherapy. More information about recurrence is given in Chapter 6 (see page 61).

HIDDEN SADNESS

Do you feel that you and your family have communicated well so far? You may be right. However, a recent study carried out by a former BACUP nurse, Hilary Plant, revealed that families received little support. In a series of interviews, Ms Plant found that families bottled up their emotions and put on a brave face because they felt the patient's needs always had to come first. She found: 'Relatives were often more distressed than the patients because they had no support. The whole focus was on the patient and there was nowhere for relatives to take their emotions.'

Ms Plant discovered that the 26 families in her study nearly all associated cancer with death, despite all the publicity about improvements in treatment and outcome. Many families were worried about how they would manage once the person with cancer died.

HOW THOSE CLOSE TO YOU CAN HELP

Talking to those who are close to us is comforting. If we have allowed a trivial problem to grow out of proportion, our nearest and dearest can cut it down to its true size. Otherwise, our imaginations can offer fertile seedbeds for small, unexpressed fears. If we keep them to ourselves they may overwhelm us.

If you can't make up your mind about something, e.g. whether to try an experimental drug, or a new, alternative therapy, airing the pros and cons will help to clarify your thoughts. Recognize that a strong, *unacknowledged* emotion will strangle communication. If your nearest and dearest is on the verge of tears, or losing sleep, you need to acknowledge that you have noticed the sadness, and share in it before you will be able to talk about anything. You may sense that that someone who wants to help feels uncomfortable. You could say, 'I realize it's difficult for you to know what to say. I know I'd find it difficult if it was the other way round. But I do want to talk about . . .'

DEALING WITH YOUR ANGER

There is a big difference between acknowledging your feelings, and expecting people to notice them from your behaviour. For instance, if you are feeling angry because your recovery is slower than you expected (or you are still asking, 'Why me?'), you may feel that people will understand why you are short-tempered and rude. They may understand, but they will certainly not want to risk getting their heads bitten off by engaging you in a deep and meaningful conversation.

Your anger is legitimate, and many people find that particular emotion boosts their fighting spirit and will to survive. But you can avoid alienating your nearest and dearest by acknowledging: 'I'm too angry to talk now', or better still, 'I'm angry today because . . .' If you are feeling bitter and discouraged, but still want to talk, you could start by apologizing for being tense and irritable and go on to explain, 'I had some bad news today', or, 'I can't stop worrying about . . .'

Beware of the temptation to present your family with a two-way loser whereby you get angry if they treat you as they always did in the past rather than acknowledging things have changed, but also get angry if you are treated as an invalid.

DEALING WITH SURE-FIRE 'CURES'

It is natural for those closest to you to look for a cure for your cancer. They may read up on your disease and develop strong ideas about the line of treatment you should follow. They are not only trying to save you, but also to re-establish their own sense of personal control over their destiny, which has been shaken by your cancer diagnosis.

You may welcome this additional advice provided you are not being pressured into an unwelcome treatment, or sent on a series of wild goose chases. Sometimes you are hit with so many different suggestions that your head starts to spin. As one cancer patient remarked bitterly: 'My friends seem to think you can pick a cancer cure up from the health food shop in the same way you pick up a lipstick from Boots.'

Each time Suzanne returned home after treatment for her pancreatic cancer, she found her husband had heard about a different 'miracle' food supplement, and expected her to change her diet totally. Suzanne said: 'At the time I could hardly eat anything – and certainly didn't want to try anything unusual. In the end it got so difficult, and we argued so much, that I had to move out. I knew he was doing it because he loved me – but I couldn't stand the pressure.'

If your family and friends take a similar approach, you may need to take quite a firm stand. You could explain that there are hundreds of unproven supplements and therapies, and you cannot be expected to try each 'flavour of the week'. It would be fair to add that, at this particular time, it is essential that you rebuild your strength, and eat foods which are palatable to you. It also seems fair to thank them for caring so much.

Unfortunately, there is always a danger that well-intentioned interference by your family and friends will start to undermine your faith in your treatment programme. If you feel this is happening you may need to tell them firmly that while you understand their good intentions, their approach is not helping you.

HELPING THEM TO HELP YOU

You can soften the blow by suggesting ways in which they can genuinely help you. Maybe you need a listening ear or would enjoy their company on an outing. Your more pragmatic friends may turn out to be useful companions on your next hospital visit, especially if you are to be presented with a lot of technical information. Finding something for helpful friends to do can be a kindness to them as much as to yourself.

After your latest hospital check-up, it may be tempting to paint a rosy picture to relieve your friends' feelings. However, such white lies will form a barrier to communication in future. If the situation is uncertain – as is so often the case with cancer – it is more helpful in the long run if you say so. There is no need to collude in other people's desire for self-deception, unless you are sure it suits your purpose.

In her book *Patient No More*, Sharon Batt, who developed breast cancer at the age of 43, wrote of her friends' attitude: 'When I try to convey the uncertainty of my prognosis, they are puzzled or incredulous. Everyone wants closure, but I am getting stubborn. I'd like closure too, but the doctors won't give it to me. And if I can't have it, I'm not about to let my friends have it either.'

If you do not have the emotional energy to deal with the fears and your anxieties of your nearest and dearest, then don't try. Some otherwise close families can be suffocating at times of crisis – and now the crisis is over you may need a break. If this is the case it may be easier to talk to colleagues or more distant family members. Sometimes people will offer the right help at the wrong time. If you don't want to think or talk about cancer now, then say so, and add that you know that you will want to talk about it another time.

AND THE NOT SO DEAR

Schadenfreude – revelling in the misfortunes of others – is an unfortunate characteristic of human nature. Some acquaintances will appear to get a grim satisfaction from chewing over your illness, and telling you about other people they have known with cancer. However badly you may have suffered, these anecdotal others will always have suffered worse. If these people are really insensitive they will add after a pause: 'Of course, it got her in the end.'

You may also be irritated to discover that some family members or acquaintances talk about you instead of to you. We all know individuals who, because of their negative attitude to life, sap our energies. If we have known them for years, or they are related to us, then they can be hard to avoid under normal circumstances. However, illness, recuperation and above all the invention of the telephone answering machine, provide an ideal refuge from not particularly well-meaning busybodies.

Suzanne, who was having a tough time coming to terms with her pancreatic cancer, explained: 'I decided that while I was feeling ill, I would treat myself by only talking to people I wanted to talk to. I left the answering machine on all the time and only returned calls to people I liked. It ran up the phone bill, but it was worth every penny.'

AND WHAT ABOUT THE KIDS?

Whatever the age of our children, there is a temptation to 'spare' them any distress. But if your adult children try to talk to your about your cancer, and you do not respond, they may well feel hurt and shut out. They can also be a great source of comfort and support and once the cancer crisis is truly over, the whole experience can draw families closer together.

For young children, your illness probably represented a period of time when both you and your partner were missing for long periods (you in hospital, and your partner working, visiting and frantically making arrangements). When life becomes 'normal' again, you can start to repair any damage or hurts caused when you were fully occupied with your illness.

You may now discover that however carefully you thought you explained the situation, your children require further information and reassurance. One way a young child expresses this need is to keep asking the same question over and over again, as he or she attempts to make sense of what happened. Be alert for the repeated question about why it happened – and be prepared to reassure the child that the illness was no one's fault.

Young children still occupy a semi-fantasy world, and can easily convince themselves that bad things happen because of their own naughty behaviour. Be sure to talk to them about what they think about your illness and correct any false impressions. Ask open questions such as, 'What would you like to know about my illness?'

While you may want to protect them from some of the details of your treatment, avoid whispered discussions behind doors which may make them feel excluded and frightened. It is understandable to want to spare your children unnecessary distress. Remember, however, that if you don't tell them, someone else will.

Margaret, 55, who has had both stomach and breast cancers,

said: 'I told my two elder children the truth about my stomach cancer, but spared the 13-year-old because I thought he would be too upset. Some kind soul at school told him, adding the information that people die of cancer. He came straight home in tears, demanding to know why I hadn't told him, and he refused to leave me. We had to get him a private tutor because he wouldn't go to school.'

If there have been changes in your body shape, or you have an operation scar, you might consider allowing the child to look or touch. A lot will depend, on course, on family attitudes to privacy and nudity. However, if a scar or body change remains hidden, the child may imagine something far worse than the reality, and his or her fear of this 'mutilation' may create barriers between you.

Cancer inevitably creates a whole range of tensions – people may bicker about trivial things to relieve their tensions about bigger issues they dare not air. Because young children believe the whole world centres on them, they may well assume that it is all their fault if the atmosphere becomes strained. As a result the child may become withdrawn and unobtrusive in the hope of putting things right or may resort to attention-seeking behaviour such as bed-wetting, whining, food refusal and disobedience. Some of this behaviour is designed to test whether you will withdraw your love from them. However, if your child behaves in an unusual and extreme way for weeks at a time, or talks of hopelessness and suicide, then you may need to call in a professional counsellor.

ADOLESCENTS

Older children may feel confused and resentful about being drawn back into the family at a time when they were working hard to establish themselves as separate individuals. They may feel torn between the desire to spend as little time as possible with an adult and terrible guilt that they don't want to be with you. This can turn to resentment, that you are laying this 'guilt trip' on them, leading in turn to more guilt.

Many adolescents are too self-absorbed to behave like adults, even in a family crisis. They are already making a point of talking to anyone but their parents (as is normal for their age), but they do need to talk to someone, and preferably an adult, about their feelings over your illness.

CHAPTER 4

DOES IT RUN IN THE FAMILY?

One of my sisters had stomach cancer and died, the other had a mastectomy and survived. I have had both types of cancer – and now I'm worried about my son, who is having stomach problems.

MARGARET, WHO HAS BEEN TREATED FOR STOMACH
AND BREAST CANCERS

FAMILY CANCERS

When someone close is diagnosed with cancer, we are all reminded of our own mortality. The reminder is all the more forcible when it becomes apparent that the type of cancer involved is inherited. It may seem bad enough to have to deal with your family's grief and anger over your cancer diagnosis. Unfortunately you may also need to address their fears – real or imagined – that the disease might run in the family.

The mysteries of genetic science are unfolding incredibly rapidly – in fact there is some concern that it may be moving rather too quickly. There are already genetic tests available for some cancers to help individuals determine their risk. Even when the gene has not been identified, scientists can compare blood samples from family members who develop cancer with those who do not. Similarities and differences in certain sections of DNA (the cell's genetic blueprint) will help to determine who is at risk and who is not.

However, genetic testing is only offered when there is a strong suspicion that a disease 'runs in the family'. Anyone considering a test should be carefully counselled to see if they are ready to deal with what could be very unwelcome and disheartening information.

Early Warning Signs of Cancer

Many cancers can be picked up early enough to avoid serious illness or death, if only symptoms are reported in time. Unfortunately, when cancer is known to run in families, people may be too frightened to report lumps and bumps and unexpected symptoms in time for an effective treatment.

Cancers are always easier to treat if they are picked up early, so your family may be interested in some of the warning signs. This list is also relevant to you, because having one type of cancer does not protect you from developing another one. And yes, some people really are that unlucky – and still survive!

Symptoms Requiring Investigation

- Rapid weight loss without apparent cause
- A scab, sore or ulcer that fails to heal after three weeks
- A blemish or mole that enlarges, bleeds or itches
- Severe recurrent headaches
- Difficulty in swallowing
- Persistent hoarseness
- Coughing up bloody sputum (phlegm)
- Persistent abdominal pain
- Change in shape and size of testes
- Blood in urine, but no pain on urination
- Change in bowel habits
- Lump or change in breast shape
- Bleeding or discharge from nipple
- Vaginal spotting or bleeding between periods or after menopause

---

If any of the symptoms shown in the box persist for more than a few days, you should visit your doctor. You may know to your cost that cancer does not always yield such handy early warnings, nevertheless if people acted on this list, many deaths could be prevented.

Avoiding Risk Factors

According to the American Cancer Society, if current knowledge about the prevention of cancer was put into practice, then up to two-thirds of cases could be avoided. The American Cancer Society says that nutrition and diet play a major role and suggests the following:

1 Maintain a desirable weight. Someone who is 40 per cent overweight, e.g. 88.9 kg (14 stones/196 lb) when they should be 63.5 kg (10 stones/140 lb) has an increased risk of colon, breast, prostate, gallbladder, ovary and womb cancers.
2 Eat a varied diet.
3 Include a variety of vegetables and fruits as this is associated with decreased risks of lung, prostate, bladder, oesophageal, colo-rectal and stomach cancers.
4 Eat more high-fibre foods such as whole-grain cereals, breads and pasta. These are a healthy substitute for fatty foods and may reduce the risk of colon cancer.
5 Cut down on total fat intake. A diet high in fat is thought to be a factor in the development of cancers of the breast, colon and prostate.
6 Limit alcohol consumption, or don't drink at all. Heavy drinking, especially when accompanied by cigarette smoking, increases the risk of cancers of the mouth, larynx, throat, oesophagus and liver.
7 Limit consumption of salt-cured, smoked and nitrite-cured foods because these have been associated with increases in cancer of the oesophagus and stomach.

In addition, the American Cancer Society advises: avoidance of smoking, which is responsible for 30 per cent of all cancer deaths; sunlight, because nearly all skin cancers are related to ultraviolet radiation from the sun; and smokeless tobacco, because chewing tobacco or the use of snuff increase the risk of cancer of the mouth, larynx, throat and oesophagus. It advocates care over the use of oestrogen in hormone replacement therapy because of the increased risk of womb cancer (in the UK, women who have not had a hysterectomy are given progestogen in their HRT to combat this risk); and warns against occupational hazards including exposure to nickel, chromate, asbestos and vinyl chloride, and ionizing radiation, in particular excess radon in the home (the risks that radon may cause lung cancer are greatly increased in smokers).

WHY ME? HOW CANCER OCCURS

The cells within our bodies are constantly multiplying. Parent cells divide to form daughter cells – exact copies of themselves. When they are no longer required, the 'old' cells are programmed to die off. It is a system that works beautifully until the genes that control cell division become faulty (mutate). This fault may be inherited, or may occur spontaneously. The reasons for this spontaneous change are not fully understood, although we do know that certain substances, known as carcinogens (e.g. tobacco smoke, radiation), can cause genetic faults.

As a result, the daughter cells cease to be exact copies of the parent. Such mistakes constantly occur, but are usually destroyed by the tumour-suppressor genes and other fail-safe mechanisms of the immune system. It is only when these safeguards fail that cells start to multiply in an uncontrolled way, forming tumours.

Even when a faulty gene is inherited, other things need to go wrong before cancer appears, otherwise everyone who inherited a cancer gene would die in early childhood. Other influences play a part, including environmental factors such as diet, radiation and exposure to chemical pollutants.

INHERITED CANCERS

Although inherited cancers can arise at any age, those which occur in younger people (the under-fifties) seem more likely to be found in families. Do not be too alarmed if you can think of more than one elderly relative who has suffered cancer. One person in three develops cancer at some stage in their lives, so it would be surprising if there were no cases in your family. The longer people survive, the greater the chances that a series of faults will occur in the fail-safe mechanisms that govern cell division. And, of course, these days people are surviving much longer.

Cancers which can show patterns of inheritance include retinoblastoma (a childhood eye cancer) and cancers of the lymph system (lymphoma), testes, breast (male and female), bowel, ovaries, skin (malignant melanoma), prostate, thyroid and brain. The search is on to identify the faulty genes in all these diseases (and in fact, some have already been located).

If you believe that cancer may run in your family, draw up a family tree to demonstrate which members are affected, and then take it to your family doctor. He or she may be able to offer immediate reassurance, or to refer you to a specialist for genetic counselling. Even then, the odds are that the geneticist will be able to reassure your that your risk is much the same as anyone else's. Only a minority of patients attending these clinics need blood tests and regular screening.

Some cancer genes appear to increase your risk slightly, and a number of other things would need to go wrong at cellular level before you developed cancer. Other genes carry a much stronger risk. For instance if you have at least three relatives with colon cancer, in two generations (at least one of whom was diagnosed before the age of 50), then you have a one in four risk of developing the disease yourself.

In families with many cases of breast cancer, the daughters of affected women may have a 50 per cent risk of inheriting the gene (which can also be passed from father to daughter). If your parent has the rare inherited form of bowel cancer, familial adenomatous polyposis (FAP), then you have a 50 per cent risk of inheriting the disease.

GENETIC SCREENING

There is no point in telling someone he or she is at increased risk of cancer, unless you can do something to help them. Genetic screening clinics offer counselling and try to give patients an accurate idea of their increased risk. They arrange for high-risk people to have regular, detailed health checks, including x-rays, colonoscopy (in the case of bowel cancer) and blood tests. Screening tests are getting better all the time, including computer-enhanced mammography for younger women (for whom ordinary mammograms can yield unsatisfactory results). Blood tests designed to detect cancer markers are also being expanded, but there are fears that gene testing is moving faster than screening, treating or curing cancer. Unfortunately, scientists often need to look for more than one faulty gene in conditions such as inherited breast cancer and colo-rectal cancer.

People vary enormously in their attitude towards genetic screening. Some high-risk individuals say that when it becomes available they will definitely have it, while others prefer not to know what is written in their genes. Patients with positive results from screening can face difficult decisions, such as whether to have their breasts or ovaries removed to prevent the development of future disease, or whether they should avoid starting a family.

People who are given the all-clear following genetic screening will obviously be tremendously relieved, and will be saved from unnecessary tests for the disease. Many people attending the clinics can be reassured. Dr Gwen Turner of the ICRF (Imperial Cancer Research Fund) family cancer clinic in Leeds commented: 'We are often able to tell people their actual risk of developing a cancer is much lower than they thought.'

However, genetic clinics cannot offer anyone a complete all-clear. Someone who is told she does not have the gene for the type of breast cancer that runs in her family still has the same risk of the disease as any other woman in the general population.

The emotional effects of a positive gene test are also worrying. Dr Caryn Lerman of the Lombardi Cancer Center at Georgetown University, Washington DC, reported testing for cancer susceptibility has a profound psychological impact. She found that the people most likely to request genetic counselling showed heightened anxiety, depression and guilt. Yet it is known that women with breast cancer who show this degree of distress are likely to avoid breast examinations and x-rays.

In the UK, of women referred for testing because of their inherited risk of breast cancer, one in four admitted that attending the clinic increased their level of anxiety. One in three showed significant levels of psychological distress when they attended the clinic and nearly one in four were people who coped by generally not seeking out further information about threatening situations. Geneticists are concerned that testing may result in cancer-susceptible people from being excluded from jobs, mortgages or life insurance.

The Nuffield Council on Bioethics in the UK warned in 1993: 'People found to be at risk from genetic disease, and their families, can face social stigma and appalling moral dilemmas about parenthood. Leaked or misinterpreted confidential genetic data could have serious lifelong consequences for an individual's employment and insurance prospects.'

Two years later, Prof. Brian Leyland-Jones of the department of clinical oncology, McGill University, Montreal, said: 'Genetic testing is not a benign intervention. Participants may require time to ponder the pros and cons, and varied strategies may be needed to approach participants of different ages.'

CHAPTER 5

Love, Sex and Relationships

After my mastectomy, my husband never saw me without my clothes on.

Breast cancer patient, 48

They told me I would still be fertile with one testicle, but I didn't really believe it until the birth of my son.

Testicular cancer patient, 39

Sexual problems

Many people are reluctant to bother their doctors about their lovemaking difficulties. They feel that they are the only ones with a problem, or that they should 'forget about that sort of thing' now that they have got cancer.

In fact, most people with cancer have difficulties with lovemaking and sexual relationships during their treatment and recovery. Anxiety, depression, worries about money and job prospects will dampen anyone's libido, regardless of whether or not they have cancer. Doctors and nurses are well aware that cancer patients have sexual problems, although sometimes embarrassment makes them reluctant to raise the issues.

It is easy to blame cancer treatment for your loss of sexual desire, when the causes are actually psychological. Equally, you may assume your loss of interest lies in the mind, when it is actually a temporary side effect. In either case, you should give your doctor the chance to correct any false beliefs. Even if your cancer unit cannot help, the medical staff should be able to refer you to someone who can. Otherwise, voluntary agencies such as

BACUP or the American Cancer Society can provide practical advice, verbally and in the form of booklets.

CELIBACY

You may, of course, have the reverse problem, where doctors and nurses are urging you to have sex when you have no wish to do so. Many people are celibate by choice, including 12 per cent of married couples. Cancer does not mean that sex suddenly becomes compulsory.

EMOTIONAL PROBLEMS

Often the reasons for sexual problems are emotional: no one feels sexy when they have gone through a painful, life-threatening experience. Drug treatments and radiotherapy can also affect the libido and make lovemaking difficult or painful.

You may find it difficult to get used to changes in your appearance such as the loss of hair, or dramatic gains or losses of weight. Some people will also have to cope with a completely different-sounding voice, following surgery to remove the voice box. Radiotherapy to the throat or larynx may have a permanent deepening effect. Any operation, even a minor one such as sterilization, can leave you feeling bruised and injured. People whose treatment is involuntary and unwelcome are likely to feel much more damaged.

The effects of cancer surgery on individual sexuality vary. Some women, for instance, accept the need for a mastectomy to increase their chances of survival. They regret the loss of the breast, but they manage to avoid being traumatized by it. Others will feel scarred and mutilated, until they can have the missing breast or breasts reconstructed with the aid of implants. One man may be philosophical about the loss of a testis and argue, correctly, that he is still as potent and fertile as anyone else. Yet another man will feel he has in some sense been 'un-manned'.

It is a natural and common reaction to be upset by the loss of any body part, even if the organ concerned is internal, and the loss is not visible or obvious. However, now you are past the 'survival at all costs' stage, you may need to repair the damage that cancer has caused to your body image, and to your relationship with your partner.

ANTIDEPRESSANTS AND LIBIDO

Anxiety and depression can reduce your desire to make love, but unfortunately some of the drugs used to treat these conditions can also interfere with your enjoyment of lovemaking. There is a wide range of antidepressant drugs on the market, and if you have this unwanted side effect, your doctor should be able to move you on to another medication which suits you better.

CHANGES IN BODY IMAGE

If someone suggested you loved your partner because of the shape of his right leg, or your daughter because of her left eyebrow, you would think it ridiculous. We are all much more than the sum of our body parts. But, of course, it is easy to say that when those parts are intact.

When you were in hospital, fighting your cancer, you may not have had the time or space to consider the possible effects of surgery on your body shape. Sometimes it can be many weeks before the implications of what has happened sink in. Coming to terms with the removal of part of your body – whether the change is internal or external – can be very difficult.

Such losses are the price cancer patients pay for the hope of longer survival and once people recover from the initial shock they generally feel it is a price worth paying. But reaching that level of acceptance takes time. As we have seen, the people who suffer most are likely to be those who torture themselves with false ideas about the reactions of others to their changed body shape.

Anger and regrets are natural, but if you are to recover well, it is important to work through these emotions and leave them behind, rather than feed them with more anger and more regret.

FEAR OF REJECTION

If people feel that they have been disfigured or have lost their attractiveness, they may 'get in first' by rejecting their partner. A man who has had a colostomy for bowel cancer may claim his treatment has left him impotent, for instance, rather than risk rejection when he tries to make love. A single woman may avoid dating rather than risk ever having to explain her hysterectomy scar. In theory the answer to such problems lies in clear and honest communication. In practice, these people will need help in accepting their changed body image and learning to love themselves again, before they can achieve it.

If you feel this applies to you, then you might try the thought-challenging techniques described in Chapter 2 (see page 20). For instance, the man could ask himself how likely it is that his wife will coldly reject him because of his colostomy bag. Attempting a closer relationship with her may give her what he wants – a closer relationship. If she really does reject him, he will be no worse off than he is now.

The woman might also consider the consequences of telling a new partner she has had cancer. If he accepts her as she is, then she would have the relationship she wants. If he rejects her, he would not be worth knowing in any case.

Some people's problems are too deep-rooted to benefit from DIY therapy. You may need one-to-one advice from a counsellor or psychotherapist based at the hospital or recommended by one of the cancer support services. To get it, you will have to admit your problem and ask for help.

FALTERING RELATIONSHIPS

Cancer can make strong marriages stronger. Each partner will recognize the true worth of the other, put petty squabbles aside, and resolve to spend more time with their loved one.

However, cancer is likely to be the last straw in a failing, or non-communicating, marriage. If you and your partner were unable to (or uninterested) in talking about your feelings, then it will be difficult to start now. Unfortunately some people who thought their marriages were reasonably solid can be bitterly disappointed by their partner's reaction to their illness. If you develop cancer and your partner walks out, it might seem like the end of the world. In the long run, you may find you thrive once you have shaken off a dead or destructive relationship. Cancer can be quite enough to contend with.

Deirdre, 47, was dismayed when her husband moved into the spare bedroom after her mastectomy. She assumed he was afraid of damaging her scar, but didn't feel she could talk to him about it. 'We didn't talk about small things – how could we talk about this?' she said.

Three years later Deirdre was still sleeping alone. 'I was terribly hurt at first. At a time when I really needed to be reassured that I was an attractive woman, he just shut me out. I think he was afraid of the cancer, and also couldn't accept the changes to my body.

'I thought I was the only one, but then I discovered two other women in my support group had been going through the same thing. In the end we agreed that we hadn't lost anything when our husbands moved into the next room. It would have been a loss if our husbands had been the kind of people who stood by us, but they weren't. I decided I was still me, just the same person, and I still had the love of my children. One thing which cancer does is to make you reassess your values.'

Lucy, who was diagnosed with cervical cancer at 44, said: 'My husband is an educated man and he knows you don't catch cancer in the same way you catch a cold. But he admitted he didn't want to make love and when I asked him about it, he admitted he was worried that he might be infected when his penis came into contact with my cervix. I understood how he felt, and I was glad he had been honest with me. I encouraged him to see our family doctor for reassurance, and that is what he did.'

RESUMING LOVEMAKING

Couples can easily fall out of the habit of lovemaking during the traumatic months of diagnosis and treatment. Each partner may assume the other one does not want sex. You may need to broach the subject in a positive way, saying: 'I do miss our lovemaking – do you think we could try again soon?' rather than a reproachful, 'It's a shame you've gone off sex.' If your sex life was once enjoyable and fulfilling, you owe it to yourself to try and regain it.

Sharon, who had a radical hysterectomy after being diagnosed with cervical cancer at 46, said: 'After the operation, I felt as if the lower half of my body was nothing to do with me. I couldn't imagine ever feeling anything in that region again. I certainly never thought I would be able to have an orgasm. When, six weeks after my surgery, I was told I could have sex again, I just laughed. But in the end I decided I would have to do it for the sake of my marriage. The first few times it was pretty uncomfortable, but it was important for us both that I tried. It was all part of feeling well again – and getting back to a normal life.'

Kevin, whose cancer treatment involved removing one testicle, said: 'I was told it wouldn't make a difference to my love life, but I was worried that I would find it difficult. I needed to prove that everything was working as it should do, before I believed what the doctors had said.'

In the BACUP booklet, *Sexuality and Cancer*, Dr Andrew Stanway, a psychosexual therapist and marital physician, suggests: 'Don't make a dash straight for intercourse . . . start slowly and gently. Try caressing one another without going for orgasm in the first few weeks. Remember that there are so many loving and erotic activities other than intercourse itself. Partners who can lovingly caress an area that has been operated upon give their partners a gift that is beyond price – the gift of acceptance. . . .

'However bad the effects of treatment, people with loving partners who can communicate with each other and explore sexually pleasurable activities can still enjoy fulfilling sex, even if what goes on in the bedroom is rather different from before.'

BACUP's Kathleen Sheridan Russell comments: 'Often cancer patients with sexual problems can't face telling their doctors face to face. If that is the problem, I suggest they call our helpline.'

SPECIAL PROBLEMS FACED BY WOMEN

HORMONAL PROBLEMS

The female hormone oestrogen is essential for female fertility and vaginal conditioning and lubrication. Many women falsely believe oestrogen also controls the libido and blame any loss of desire on a treatment-induced menopause. In fact the hormones which fuel female desire are androgen – weak forms of the male hormones. Androgens are produced from the adrenal glands at the top of the kidneys.

If your ovaries are removed or inactivated, your hormones will be in disarray and you may not feel very sexy for a while. But if you go off sex for good, you need to investigate causes other than the loss of oestrogen. Having said that, loss of oestrogen does make lovemaking difficult because the vagina remains tight and dry, even when a woman is aroused. You may also find yourself going through an intense, speeded-up menopause; see section on loss of fertility (page 55).

EFFECTS OF RADIOTHERAPY

Radiotherapy to the vagina and cervix (neck of the womb) may cause scarring and loss of elasticity. Radiotherapy can also reduce the natural secretions, thus making the vagina feel tight and dry. You may have been advised to resume lovemaking as soon as possible to help to keep the tissues stretched, although if you are still shocked by your diagnosis this may be the last thing on your mind.

Failing that, or if you do not have a partner, you can keep the tissues flexible with the aid of vaginal dilators (your doctor should be able to advise on this). Alternatively you could try gently stretching the vagina each evening, beginning with one well-lubricated finger, and then progressing to two or more. Some women who have had reconstructive surgery to the vagina will need to use dilators continuously at first, and then three times a week for life.

Radiation to the pelvic area often affects the ovaries and may cause temporary or permanent sterility. Sex is perfectly safe during radiotherapy, but you should protect yourself against pregnancy.

EFFECTS OF CHEMOTHERAPY

If you face chemotherapy in future, and are still fertile, you will need to take precautions against pregnancy. Many chemotherapy drugs can be extremely harmful to a developing fetus. See section on infertility (page 57).

EFFECTS OF SURGERY

Surgery on the vagina, or on the delicate area between the vagina and the anus, may cause pain during intercourse. In this situation, lovemaking should be started very gradually, possibly without penetration, for several weeks. Penetrative sex may be easier if the woman lies on top of her partner, or sideways so that she can more easily withdraw if intercourse becomes painful.

During a hysterectomy, the top of the vagina is stitched. While this scar is healing, it may be easier to avoid penetrative sex or find different positions. Some women find that their experience of orgasm is less intense after a hysterectomy because of the loss of sensations caused by the rhythmic contractions of the womb.

Some women who have had mastectomies will prefer a change of position in which they are lying on top, or to the side of their partner. Some will choose to wear a prosthesis or camisole top in bed, while others may enjoy being touched round the site of the scar. Many women find their partners are much less upset by mastectomy scars than they expected.

BREAST RECONSTRUCTION

If you are unhappy about your new shape, you can ask to be referred to a plastic surgeon to discuss breast reconstruction. Although sensations in the reconstructed breast will never be the same as in the other breast, some women find reconstruction makes a vast difference to their self-image.

Reconstruction surgery is not always successful. Implants may occasionally cause rejection problems, and need to be removed. Removal may also be necessary if, as sometimes happens, they become surrounded by a capsule of hard scar tissue.

LOSS OF FERTILITY

Any treatment that affects a woman's ovaries may cause symptoms of an early menopause, e.g. missing or irregular periods, hot flushes, night sweats, dry skin and vaginal dryness. This artificial menopause can produce sudden, strong symptoms that cause a great deal of misery, at a time when your self-esteem is likely to be at rock bottom.

This sudden 'change' can be caused by radiotherapy, surgical removal of the ovaries, chemotherapy or the hormonal drug, tamoxifen. Unfortunately, some of the most commonly used chemotherapy drugs, including methotrexate and melphalan are most likely to produce such symptoms. If this happens to you, do ask the doctor in charge of your treatment if the effects are likely to be permanent, or if (as is occasionally possible) a hormone treatment may bring your fertility back to normal.

Such treatments are not the same as hormone replacement therapy (HRT), which is often given to women who became infertile after treatment. HRT will relieve the symptoms of the menopause, and also protect you against the future risks of osteoporosis and heart disease, but it will not get your ovaries working again. Your doctor may find that you need a slightly larger than normal dose of HRT to control your symptoms. If you have had a hysterectomy, you will only need oestrogen, but women whose wombs are intact are nearly always prescribed oestrogen and progestogen therapy.

HRT used to be considered unsafe for women with breast cancer. Some doctors now feel the benefits outweigh any possible risks, although the nature of your tumour is likely to influence the final decision (some breast cancers are hormone-dependent).

There is, as yet, no consensus among doctors about whether it is safe to prescribe HRT for cancer patients. The uncertainty over this issue means that one doctor may agree to your request for hormone replacement, while another may say that he or she does not think it is a good idea. HRT is generally considered unsafe for women who have endometrial cancer, or have had adenocarcinoma of the cervix.

SPECIAL PROBLEMS FACED BY MEN

HORMONAL PROBLEMS

Until fairly recently, men with advanced prostate cancer had their testes removed, or were given female hormones to slow the progress of the disease. These days an injection is given to stop the pituitary gland from producing male hormones, along with hormone-blocking tablets. The effects are the same, and work as well in controlling the cancer, as testicular surgery. This hormone treatment always causes infertility, and often leads to a decreased sex drive.

EFFECTS OF RADIOTHERAPY

Radiotherapy treatment for cancers of the prostate, rectum and bladder sometimes cause difficulties with erection. This is because of damage to the nerves or blood vessels that supply the penis. This problem, which affects about one treated man in three, can be a delayed after-effect that appears many months after treatment has finished. A few men may also notice a reduced sex drive caused by radiation affecting the testicles.

EFFECTS OF CHEMOTHERAPY

This seldom has lasting effects on the male sex drive. If you believe your chemotherapy has interfered with your ability to make love, check first with your doctor. It may be that your problems are psychological, or have some non-drug-related cause. Avoid making your partner pregnant while you are on chemotherapy, because the drugs can cause abnormalities in sperm.

EFFECTS OF SURGERY

Surgery on the prostate or rectum may lead to altered sensations of ejaculation, or affect the nerves that control sexual functioning. You may notice a dry orgasm, where sex is still pleasurable, but the semen goes into the bladder and is discharged from the body when you next urinate. A good flow of blood needs to enter the penis to produce an erection. Surgery may sometimes interfere with the nerves controlling the blood vessels that supply the penis.

TREATMENTS FOR IMPOTENCE

Don't be too quick to write off your sex life. Some men find the effects of surgical damage wear off in time, and they are able to resume normal sexual activity. Others blame their surgery for problems that lie in the mind (and if recognized, are easier to correct than many physical problems). Erection difficulties can sometimes be remedied with surgery to improve the blood flow in the penis, or with penile implants or injections.

PERFORMANCE ANXIETY

Many of the effects of cancer on sexuality are temporary. Unfortunately, it is easy to give up in embarrassment if lovemaking has failed once or twice. Men are particularly vulnerable to this type of performance anxiety. If you have tried and failed to make love since your diagnosis, it may well be time to try again.

LOSS OF FERTILITY

The most commonly used chemotherapy drugs interfere with the way the cells reproduce, and can cause infertility in men. Radiotherapy to the testes can produce temporary or permanent infertility because it interferes with production of the male hormone, testosterone.

Surgical operations including abdomino-perineal resection for colo-rectal cancer can sometimes cause infertility while removal of the prostate or both testes always does. In some cases sperm can be removed before the procedure, stored and used to inseminate the man's partner later.

CHAPTER 6

Dealing with the Unexpected

And that which I am afraid of cometh unto me,
I am not at ease, neither am I quiet, neither have I rest;
But trouble cometh.

Job 3:25

Delayed after-effects

You can be tremendously brave and stoical, only to find yourself knocked off course by something entirely unexpected. It may be a recurrence, just as you thought you were out of the woods, or a delayed after-effect of treatment. And, of course, it might turn out to be a genuine ailment which has nothing to do with your cancer. You are as likely to get arthritis, or a strained muscle, backache or neckache from sitting in a draught as anyone else. Yet understandably many people think of cancer if a new or unexpected symptom occurs.

Danny, 41, had been successfully treated for a recurrence of his testicular teratoma. Two years later, he started to feel lethargic, and felt a tight band across his chest as he got out of bed and one of his feet swelled up. The cardiologist could find no sign of heart damage, so Danny was referred back to his cancer specialist.

'I thought the cancer had come back and I felt frustrated and sad. Things had been going so well, my wife was expecting a baby, and I just wanted to get on with my life. I think the doctors at the hospital assumed it was cancer as well.' However, tests showed no sign that the cancer had recurred, and after several weeks of uncertainty for Danny, a rheumatologist was called in. 'He knew what it was immediately as soon as I described my symptoms. He said I was a textbook case of ankylosing spondylitis.'

Danny says the condition, which is caused by inflammation of the joints between the vertebrae, causes more problems than his cancer. 'People ask me about my cancer, but my back is much more of a nuisance. With the cancer, you zap it and it goes away, and you can forget about it. With this, it can flare up at any time.'

New symptoms can also signal a delayed after-effect of treatment. Fifteen years after his experimental chemotherapy saved his life, Danny started to notice that he could no longer hear high tones. This was the first sign that his platinum treatment had actually damaged his hearing nerves. Danny is philosophical: 'I go with the flow. My treatment saved my life at a time when doctors had only given me a few weeks to live.'

Doctors and nurses find it difficult to decide how much they should tell patients about some of the rarer and more serious side effects that might occur. The booklets issued by hospitals and cancer charities sometimes omit this information, rather than risk upsetting patients unnecessarily. Unfortunately, this lack of knowledge can sometimes lead people falsely to assume their disease has recurred. Even if you are warned of an unpleasant after-effect, bear in mind the fact that it might not occur. For example, after Margaret's stomach was removed, she was told she would have to live on a diet of babyfood. After a few months, she was bored stiff, and cautiously reintroduced normal food into her diet. She found that she could eat much the same diet as her husband and friends, although in much smaller quantities.

Likewise, Renée was warned that her arm might be paralysed after surgery to her neck and shoulder. 'When the surgeon came to see me after the operation, I raised my arm into the air. There is some loss of flexibility, but it still works.'

This chapter, along with Chapters 10 and 11 (see pages 123 and 134), aims to give a frank idea of some of the immediate and late side effects of treatment. Some of the symptoms and after-effects described are quite rare, and most will not affect you personally. If you are having a treatment for the first time, or require further treatment, you will find more information in Chapters 10 and 11 (see pages 123 and 134).

LYMPHOEDEMA

The sudden swelling of an arm or leg months or years after cancer treatment is very common – and yet many people complain they were not warned that this could happen to them. It is caused when the body's natural drainage system is damaged by surgery or radiotherapy. It affects the arms of women whose breast cancer treatment has involved surgery or radiotherapy in the armpit, and the legs of people who have been treated in the pelvic region (usually for cancer of the cervix, bowel or prostate).

Lymph is a colourless fluid, containing white blood cells, proteins and fats, which plays an important role in the body's natural defence system. Lymphoedema is often triggered by an infection, and the cause can be as trivial as a scratch from a rose thorn. Fluid builds up in the surrounding tissues, causing pain and swelling.

Sally, 55, who developed lymphoedema after a hysterectomy for cervical cancer said: 'The sensation of your limb filling with fluid is like cold ants crawling up your leg. The skin gets tighter, and the limb becomes so heavy that it is hard to step up a kerbstone or climb stairs.'

Sally's swollen legs signalled a breakdown in her body's natural drainage channels – the lymphatic system. Her lymphoedema was triggered by a mosquito bite while she was on holiday in Spain. At first her condition was mistaken for thrombosis and when this was ruled out, she was prescribed diuretics (water pills), which proved ineffective. Sally, a slim choreographer, was distressed to find her lower half was a UK size 14, (US size 12) while her top was a UK size ten (US size 8). It was only after reading about similar symptoms in a newspaper article that she realized that her problem was a delayed side effect of her cancer treatment.

She says: 'If I had known that I was at risk of lymphoedema, I could have taken antibiotics immediately when the insect bite became infected. That would have given me a good chance of keeping the condition under control. Better still, I could have used insect repellents and worn long trousers to reduce my risk. As it was, I was left plodding around on vast legs.

'When I finally found someone to help me, I couldn't believe that I was really going to have to wear these dreadful, ginger-coloured compression tights for the rest of my life. It was the only time that I'd actually cried over my cancer. I felt so sorry for myself, and then I decided to do something about it.' Sally became a founder member of the Lymphoedema Support Network.

Meanwhile Sally tried dyeing the tights, but discovered that there was a slight loss of elasticity. She compromised by wearing dyed tights in the evenings if she was going out. She also devised her own programme of exercise, which she carries out for 35 minutes at least three times a week. She says: 'Now the two halves of my body match, but I know that I have to wear the stockings and take special care for the rest of my life.'

If you are at risk of lymphoedema, you should try to avoid getting the vulnerable arm or legs infected. It is important to persist with any exercises the hospital has taught you to minimize the swelling, even if these seem pointless at the time. If you think you have developed lymphoedema, you should contact your local cancer unit. Some hospitals now run clinics to treat this complication, or can refer you somewhere else if necessary. Untreated lymphoedema can develop into elephantiasis – a disabling condition with massive swelling, and thickening of the skin. The self-help measures on page 65 are recommended by the Lymphoedema Support Network.

The most common treatment for lymphoedema is a specially designed elastic support sleeve or stocking, which has to be prescribed by your local hospital. Your family doctor should be able to contact the hospital on your behalf. Manual lymphatic drainage, a special kind of massage, is another important treatment, which has to be given by a trained person. Information is available from the Lymphoedema Support Network, BACUP or the American Cancer Society (see Useful Addresses, page 147).

DELAYED EFFECTS OF RADIOTHERAPY

Tiredness often affects people during radiotherapy, but fatigue can be a late effect, occurring months after your treatment. People who have had radiotherapy to the brain or total body irradiation before a bone marrow transplant may experience a condition known as somnolence syndrome a month or two after treatment has ended. This leads to feelings of tiredness, lethargy and depression, where everything seems to be too much trouble. The symptoms should disappear after about a week.

Radiotherapy to the mouth can make you susceptible to tooth decay, and you need to alert your dentist to this possibility and take his or her advice about how often you will need a check-up. You may find that the dry mouth symptoms you encountered

SELF-HELP FOR THOSE AT RISK OF LYMPHOEDEMA

- When gardening, wear gloves, long sleeves and long trousers
- Be particularly careful with sharp knives
- If your skin is cut or scratched, wash the affected area thoroughly and apply an antiseptic cream. If redness, swelling, or a boil develops, let your family doctor know as soon as possible
- If you need an injection, or want to give blood, or to have your blood pressure checked, offer the arm which is not likely to be affected
- When shaving, use an electric razor or creams rather than razor blades
- Use nail clippers rather than scissors to avoid nicking fingers or toes
- Avoid sudden strenuous movements with the affected arm, or carrying heavy shopping – but otherwise try to use the limb normally, as muscle activity helps the natural drainage
- If your leg is affected, avoid standing still for long periods
- Protect yourself against sunburn with high-factor sunscreens
- Use insect repellents, and tell your family doctor if an insect bite becomes infected
- Use moisturizers to prevent your skin from becoming dry or cracked
- Try not to become overweight because obesity may interfere with lymph drainage
- Be aware that occasionally doctors may mistake your symptoms for thrombosis

during treatment also persist. If this is the case, you could ask your doctor to prescribe an artificial saliva spray.

Several months after radiotherapy to your chest, you may be alarmed to discover you are developing a dry cough or shortness of breath. Although you should alert your doctor, this is likely to be a late symptom of radiotherapy.

Radiotherapy can also cause the breast to become firmer and harder. The skin in the treated area is often slightly darker, and the pores may be enlarged and more noticeable. Sometimes the treated breast becomes larger because of a build-up of fluid. Occasionally the breast shrinks, although this was a commoner problem in the past when doses tended to be higher and spread over a wider area. Some women who have been treated for breast cancer have developed arm weakness because of nerve damage caused by radiotherapy, although radiotherapists say this is a rare complication.

Even if you believe changes in the appearance of your breast are caused by radiation, do point them out next time you see the doctor – and, if in doubt, make a special appointment. Skin which has been irradiated is very sensitive to the effects of the sun, so you need to cover up or use effective sunscreens for at least a year.

Radiotherapy is very effective for cancers of the cervix, womb, bladder and prostate. Unfortunately some of the nearby organs, such as the liver, bowel and kidney can easily be damaged – and sometimes are. Severe side effects such as pain and bleeding can occur if organs adhere to each other, leading the patient to fear the cancer has returned. If the damage cannot be repaired, the patient may need to have a colostomy (for faeces) and urinary diversion (for urine).

Sylvia was treated with external and internal radiotherapy after being diagnosed with cervical cancer at 47. She says: 'I was fine for two years, and then I started feeling very sick. I couldn't keep food down, and I had griping pains in my stomach, I was bleeding from the bladder and my bowel wasn't working properly. I looked anorexic and the bowel specialist couldn't tell me what was wrong.

'I was frantic with worry and sure the cancer had come back. I asked to be referred back from the local hospital to the Christie Hospital in Manchester, which had treated my cancer. There the professor told me I would need major surgery and would probably end up needing a colostomy and a urine bag.

'I felt I was the unluckiest person in the world. When they took me to the operating theatre, I thought I wouldn't be the same person when I woke up. When I came round, I felt around my abdomen but there were no bags. The next morning the professor came and told me my problems had been caused by the internal radiotherapy treatment I'd had. As a result my bowel had become so thin that food could not pass through, and my bladder had been stuck to my womb. He had removed the scar tissue and repaired my bowel. The cancer hadn't come back after all.'

Unfortunately, that was not the end of it. The complex repair operation meant that Sylvia could eat again and start to put on weight. But she continued to suffer from constant diarrhoea. One day she realized, to her horror, that stools were leaking into her vagina.

'Once again I thought the cancer had come back, but my family doctor instantly knew what was wrong – and my specialist confirmed it. I had a fistula – a passage had opened from my bowel into my vagina. I needed a long operation to cut it out, and to establish a colostomy.

'I was terribly disappointed, but in fact my life is easier now. Even before the fistula appeared it had been really difficult to go out, because I could never move far from a loo. I needed vitamin injections every few weeks. The colostomy has made my life much more normal.

'The doctors have been honest and admitted all these problems were caused by my radiotherapy. But if I developed cancer again, I would have the same treatment. Without it, I wouldn't be here now.'

Another serious but rare complication of radiotherapy is axillary tunnel damage. This affects people who have had radiotherapy above the collar bone or in the armpit (and particularly women whose underarm lymph nodes are treated for breast cancer). This can cause tissue and nerve damage that can trigger tingling of the fingers, pains in the shoulder and weakness in the hand. The most serious type of damage, brachial plexopathy, can lead to paralysis of the muscles of the shoulder, elbow and forearm. These symptoms can be permanent, and need to be treated by pain specialists, physiotherapists and occupational therapists. A leaflet on the delayed effects of radiotherapy is available from BACUP (see Useful Addresses, page 147).

DELAYED EFFECTS OF DRUG THERAPIES

Doctors try hard to ensure that drug treatments designed to help patients do not cause more harm than good. Unfortunately, the difference between the dose that will destroy cancer cells and the dose that may seriously damage organs can be small. When drugs are new, doctors are not always certain of the correct dose to use (which is one reason why they are initially tested on patients for whom all other treatments have failed).

Sometimes, when a life is at stake, there is no time to wait for something better. The doctor and patient must then weigh up the risks together, and decide on how to progress. However, even well-established drugs can cause damage, and for unknown reasons, some people are more susceptible than others. Any treatment which is powerful enough to damage cancer cells may also be powerful enough to cause lasting damage.

A minority of unlucky individuals are left with lifetime side effects, such as damage to the heart, lung and kidneys. Permanent loss of sensation in the hands or feet (peripheral neuropathy) can also occur, and in extreme cases the results can be disabling. Hearing can also be affected, with the loss of high tones. Or you may avoid these hazards, but find you are constantly in the dentist's surgery because chemotherapy has made you more susceptible to tooth decay.

As described in the previous chapter, treatment can sometimes have lasting effects on sexual potency and fertility. The long-term use of corticosteroid drugs can cause osteoporosis (loss of density to the bones), which increases the risk that a minor fall or sudden movement may lead to a fracture. If you are worried about the long-term effects of your cancer drugs, ring the BACUP helpline number (see page 147) for verbal and written advice.

CANCER TREATMENTS THAT CAUSE CANCER

When combined with radiotherapy, prolonged use of the class of drugs known as alkylating agents can damage white cell production, occasionally causing leukaemia. Doctors have to balance this risk against the likelihood of an earlier death from cancer.

TREATMENTS THAT GO WRONG

Once the initial cancer emergency is over, your doctor may offer you surgery to improve your appearance, or repair any damage caused by the treatment itself. But reconstruction surgery, like any other type of operation, can go wrong.

Jane, diagnosed with breast cancer at 46, said: 'I was really excited about having a new breast after my mastectomy. My temporary implant had been removed, and a permanent one inserted. I thought it was only a matter of time before I got over the slight tautness and discomfort.

'On the day I was due to have my stitches removed, I woke up with a temperature and felt as if I'd got flu. I rang the hospital to put them off, but they insisted I came in at once. They took one look at me and admitted me on to the ward. I drifted in and out of sleep with a raging temperature and a measle-like rash spread over my breast, trunk and armpit. My breast was swollen and unbearably tight, and I felt very ill.

'On my second night in hospital, I felt a burning pain and a sensation of wetness. My stitches had burst open, and it turned out that abscesses had formed round the implant. It had to be removed, leaving me lopsided again.

'A friend of mine had the same operation and is very happy with the result, but unfortunately my body had rejected the silicone. Somehow it seemed worse to lose a breast the second time round, and I was terribly upset. But then I decided that the important thing was that I had survived my cancer. I got the latest type of prosthesis, and I make a point of choosing pretty underwear. I don't think about implants at all any more.'

FURTHER TREATMENT

Just as you thought you were out of the woods, you may find that your doctor recommends further treatment. It may be history repeating itself, with a return to a familiar drug, or more often, it is something quite different, for which you are not prepared.

If it has been several years since your first lot of therapy, you may be pleasantly surprised by the improvement in treatments. One cancer specialist invited some ex-patients along to admire his new chemotherapy unit, but found that none of them wanted to come. They all had vivid memories of months of nausea, diarrhoea and vomiting. Yet this doctor, and the staff of his new unit, pride themselves on the effective use they make of the latest anti-emetic treatments to help avoid such severe side effects.

Margaret's life was saved by chemotherapy drugs at a time when doctors expected her to die within three months of her stomach cancer. But the treatment, given for two and a half years, made her very sick and constantly needing to run to the lavatory. 'I decided then that whatever happened, I would never have chemotherapy again,' she said.

Fourteen years later she developed breast cancer. 'I felt quite differently. I realized how the drugs had helped me last time, and so I was prepared to go through it all again.' The drugs made her so nauseous that she was retching as she talked to her specialist.

'Why didn't you tell us this was making you so ill?' he enquired. Margaret explained that she thought feeling rotten was the price she had to pay. The doctor then prescribed one of the newer anti-sickness treatments, along with other medicines to relieve her symptoms. Chemotherapy was still no bed of roses, and Margaret lost her hair for the second time, but the treatment was much more bearable than on the previous occasion.

Margaret has noticed a great improvement in the amount of information given to patients, both by doctors and by the cancer charities. These days, if you want to know more about your disease, you can obtain a free booklet from one of the cancer charities (see Useful Addresses, page 147). These are written in patient-friendly language rather than medical jargon. If you want to know about research in your particular cancer, information is available from the Imperial Cancer Research Fund and the Cancer Research Campaign – or, again, from the American Cancer Society.

Doctors are now more aware of quality-of-life issues. Some familiar cancer treatments have now been fine-tuned to minimize the unpleasant effects they have on patients. However, all this does not mean that cancer therapy is any less aggressive. The use of transplants of bone marrow and peripheral blood stem cells means that cancer-killing drugs can now be given in much higher doses. At the same time, research is under way to see if giving more frequent doses of radiotherapy may improve the cancer patient's chances of survival.

HOW CANCER TREATMENTS WORK

Despite the advances which have been made – and the cures that are now being achieved – we do not know how to stop the cancer process at its genesis, when cell division and repair mechanisms start to fail. All the treatments currently available are designed to remove, starve or destroy abnormal cells that have already started to multiply. And any treatment that is strong enough to be effective against malignant cells inevitably has the capacity to do harm as well.

Most cancer treatments are tough on the patient and you will need to muster all your psychological and physical reserves if you are to benefit (see Chapters 8 and 9, pages 93 and 108). If one type of drug does not work for you, then you may be offered another. Regular blood tests will be taken to check that your therapy is not damaging vital organs, or reducing your resistance to infection to unacceptable levels.

The side effects of cancer therapies often cause a loss of appetite, at a time when your doctors and family are urging you to keep up your strength. Ideas about how to deal with the symptoms appear in Chapters 9 and 10 (see pages 108 and 123).

If you are concerned about the quality of cancer treatment you are being offered, consult Chapter 7 (see page 76) for how to get the best out of the system.

The information on treatments given in Chapters 10 and 11 (see pages 123 and 134) applies equally to newly diagnosed cancer patients who are awaiting their first lot of treatment. As you read through it, do remember that there is a wide variation in the side effects caused by drugs, and the effects of your treatment might be much milder than those described below. Many of the symptoms described here will never affect you.

Cancer treatments can make you feel quite ill and very disheartened and it is easy to forget that the point of the exercise is to make you better. Try to keep your final objective in mind at all times. Before you embark on any course of therapy you should discuss it fully with the doctor or nurse who is treating you.

Questions to Ask Before Treatment

- What are the likely side effects?
- Are there likely to be any long-term effects?
- What complications might occur that would necessitate alerting the doctor?

RECURRENCE

Cancer patients are naturally fearful that the disease will come back. Although everyone gets backache, indigestion and odd aches and pains, the cancer patient will consider, if only fleetingly, whether this is 'it'.

In fact, the reverse view is more logical. There are far more false alarms about recurrence than actual instances when cancer recurs. If your symptoms persist, and you get them checked out, the chances are that you will be reassured.

Sometimes, of course, cancer does recur, either at or near the site where it first appeared (local recurrence) or as a secondary or metastasis in a different part of the body (distant recurrence). No matter how far away it is from the original site, it is still the same cancer. Thus a breast cancer that recurs in the spine still behaves like breast cancer and responds to the treatments which work best for breast cancer.

Some cancers will never recur, some will come back within weeks or months, and some will reappear 10 or 20 years later. Understandably, many people experience sickened disappointment when they realize their cancer is back. A recurrence means the cancer is still in your body, and that you need more treatment. The chemotherapy drug which worked so well last time might achieve the same results.

Often, however, doctors find they need to treat the cancer with different drug combinations, or different types of drugs, such as hormones.

There is a limit to how much radiotherapy a body can take in a lifetime, and if your radiation treatment was intensive last time, a different approach will be needed. Surgery, which may have got rid of all visible traces of disease previously, is less effective when there are several secondaries.

You may feel so angry that you are tempted not to seek treatment at all. No one can make you have treatment which you do not want, and it is up to you to decide what is right. However, recurrence does not mean your cancer has won, and your life is now at an end. Many people are successfully treated after their cancer recurs, and even if they succumb to the disease in the end, have years more of fruitful life. Many older patients with recurrence survive to die of completely different causes.

Understandably, some people are reluctant to tell their nearest and dearest that their cancer has recurred, and try to carry the burden alone. But although this may spare them pain in the short term, friends and relatives may feel bitterly hurt later – and also regret all the things which were left unsaid because they were unaware of the true situation.

Another problem is that when you feel in need of support and affection you are unable to ask for it. Sometimes your doctor or cancer nurse can help break the news and also put the situation in perspective. Recurrence is bad news, but people can live with recurring cancer for years.

In fact some people find it helpful to think of their cancer as a long-standing condition: for most of the time they are well, but every so often it flares up.

This was the approach taken by Anne, who was told at the age of 27 that she had a couple of years to live at the most. Her breast cancer had spread to her spine and the pelvis by the time it was diagnosed, and she was told it was too late for a mastectomy.

Some types of breast cancer shrink if they are deprived of female hormones. This applied to Anne's cancer, and so her ovaries were removed, bringing on an early menopause, but halting the damage to her spine and pelvis.

In the years which followed, Anne had a number of secondary recurrences. These are generally more difficult to treat than cancers that recur on the original site, but Anne's particular form of cancer proved responsive to a variety of treatments. Anne said: 'After my ovaries were removed it was a question of taking pot shots at the cancer each time it cropped up. I had radiotherapy to my breast, underarm, shoulder, spine and pelvis. I was on chemotherapy for eight years. There were some deposits on my bladder, and one in my brain, but they were dealt with too. When one treatment didn't work, the specialist tried another.

'I carried on working although I never planned a career because I hadn't expected to last so long. When I was 41, I chose to take early retirement and have some time for myself.

'My radiotherapy didn't affect me, apart from some skin soreness like sunburn. The only effect from all that chemotherapy was that for a while I lost my hair and toenails.

'I hate fuss and I have never let people fuss over me. I don't think my cancer will ever completely go away, but I'm getting a great deal out of my life.' Anne realized that medical advances had saved her life on many occasions. She helped the fund-raising efforts of the Imperial Cancer Research Fund, acting as an inspiration to other patients.

She died 19 years after her original diagnosis, when her cancer invaded her liver. By that time her husband, Tony, had started to believe the cancer would never beat her. Anne had taken a more realistic view, but felt she had won the battle by surviving for so much longer than anyone could have expected.

Danny had a recurrence of his testicular teratoma 12 years after it was first treated, and needed to have a testicle removed. He said: 'I'd had my annual check-up in January and been told everything was fine. Within a month, in the February, my testicle had trebled in size. However, I felt fit and well, and that gave me confidence. I remembered how ill I had felt when my cancer was first diagnosed. I felt strong enough to fight it.

'That was five years ago, and apart from a false alarm when I had a spinal condition, I've been well ever since. Cancer taught me, and the recurrence reminded me, that life is short and made me want to cram as much into it as I can. I take a fatalistic view. There are certain things you can do. I avoid smoking, try to keep fit and eat a vegetarian diet. But there's no point in worrying about things you can't change, and so I don't worry about the cancer.'

For most of us, dealing with a recurrence will be even more challenging than dealing with the original diagnosis. Even if you worked hard to keep yourself in the best possible health, you may now wonder if you should have done more. However, it is important for your continuing recovery that you do not attempt to blame yourself.

Be clear in your mind that the return of cancer has a biological cause, not an emotional one. It results from changes that are taking place within the cells of your body. It has not happened because you failed to meditate, visualize, eat enough fibre, or think enough positive thoughts. Effective self-help as described in Chapter 10 (see page 93) is a powerful tool that will enable you to face up to this challenge. But it is not a weapon that cancer patients should use against themselves: cancer is quite enough to contend with.

Further treatment is often available to deal with a recurrence. However, sometimes the doctor has to admit that no further curative treatment is available, and that it is now time to concentrate on treatments to relieve your symptoms. If this is unacceptable, then you may want to consider trying a new treatment which is currently being evaluated. Very occasionally such treatments save a patient's life against all the odds: usually they don't. Information on clinical trials is given in Chapter 7 (see page 76).

CHAPTER 7

GETTING THE BEST OUT OF THE SYSTEM

*My first thought on finding I had breast cancer was
that I would never get a job again.*

DEBBIE

WORKING THE SYSTEM

You cannot make the best of your recovery if you are worried about keeping a roof over your head, or about the possibility that your doctors are not doing everything they can for you. This chapter is about how to 'work the system' to help you avoid or minimize these anxieties.

The chapter has a recurring theme: if you have a financial or medical worry, act on it immediately. Because cancer is such a common disease, there are a host of experts 'out there' who probably have the answer to your problem. They won't know about you, so it is up to you to find them. Agonizing in private is not only unproductive – it can delay your recovery.

MONEY MATTERS

Cancer does not just have implications for your health: it can have an enormous impact on your personal finances, and the consequences can linger on, long after your treatment has been completed. Unfortunately, you need to be prepared for some initial rejections when you try to put your finances in order. It will not take the disappointment away, but at least it will save you from being knocked off balance.

Insurance companies make their money by sharing risks – but they also take care to minimize their own risks of paying out. If you already had life assurance when you were diagnosed with cancer, you continue to be covered (provided you did not conceal any relevant medical information). However, you will probably find it difficult or impossible to increase the size of the policy for some years to come.

If you do not have life assurance, and your treatment was in the last year or so, the company may want to postpone acceptance for two to three years, and then charge you a hefty premium. Some types of cancer tend to recur within two or three years of diagnosis. If you have this type of cancer, and a longer period of time has passed, your chances of getting life assurance are better. Even if one company rejects you, then you will often find another that will say 'yes'.

If you do not want to shop around yourself, the British Insurance and Investment Brokers Association (BIIBA, see page 148) should be able to find you a broker. Some travel insurance companies will only insure your possessions and not your health while you are away from home. However, BIIBA can help arrange Travel Special Needs Insurance. Finally, BIIBA can provide a list of local independent financial advisors if you are finding it difficult to get a mortgage. Again, your chances of success will depend on the type and extent of your cancer, and the time since treatment.

In the US, problems can arise when insurance companies do not want to pay the full costs of your treatment. This may simply be because they are unaware of treatments, or because they are trying to limit costs. The important thing is not to panic. Many cancer patients have gone down this particular road before you. Sometimes these difficulties can be resolved by getting your physician to provide more details about the treatment to your insurance company. If this fails, then contact the Association of Community Cancer Centers (see page 149).

EMERGENCY FINANCIAL HELP

If you are in serious financial difficulties as a result of your cancer, you should ask to see your hospital social worker (if you are still receiving treatment), or contact your local social services department and ask to see a social worker.

The social worker will not only be able to advise you, but will also be able to act as your advocate in your dealings with the outside world, e.g. with the housing department, or the finance company that is funding your mortgage.

Your local Citizens Advice Bureau should be able to advise you on state benefits, and on allowances for help with mobility, care, and with fares to the hospital. You may also qualify for free prescriptions.

The Cancer Relief Macmillan Fund provides grants for home helps, home nursing, fares, holidays, heating, clothing, bedding, relatives' bed and breakfast costs, telephone installation and bills. Your community nurse or social worker will apply on your behalf, although grants are not given to people who have substantial savings.

Actors, bank employees, doctors, musicians, nurses, printers, social workers, members of the armed forces and teachers all have special benevolent funds that can help with cash grants and sometimes holidays as well. Unions and certain professional organizations may also have funds for these purposes.

In the US, you can find out about community services that might help you or relevant benevolent funds by calling your local American Cancer Society. Services which are often available include home health care, family service or counselling, transportation, help for senior citizens, assistance with money matters and job retraining. Some services have a sliding scale of fees based on your income.

EMPLOYMENT

There is tremendous variation among individuals as to how quickly they can get back to work. Cancer is not a single disease, and individuals can react to various treatments in very different ways. Some people suffer from disabling nausea and diarrhoea, while others on the same treatment may be much luckier.

A cancer diagnosis upsets all your plans and expectations, and many people need time to ground themselves again before they can think about work. And yet going back to the daily grind can be an important marker of your return to normality. It brings back some of the structure that was missing from your week, allows you to feel that you are controlling your destiny again, and, of course, it should resolve some of your financial worries.

Debbie, diagnosed with breast cancer at 43, said: 'I worked through my treatment and that was the right decision for me. It didn't stop me from thinking about my cancer – it was constantly on my mind. Nine months after it was diagnosed, I got a new job and felt that I could look forward again. It proved to me that as far as my work was concerned, nothing had changed.'

Not everyone has Debbie's strong urge to continue 'business as usual'. Many people find their attitude to work has changed. It is not that your job has become less interesting, but simply that the rest of your life has become more interesting. The months after treatment become an opportunity to reconsider what is really important to you.

John's surgery and chemotherapy for bowel cancer made him quite ill, but also gave him time to reflect. He said: 'I realized that I had been ill for some time before my cancer was diagnosed, but I was trying to open another regional office and ignoring what my body was telling me. One thing I've learned is a better idea of when to stop.

'My employer was very good. I was on full pay for six months, and half pay for the seventh month, when I went back. I also went into the office a couple of times during my chemotherapy to test the water. I am still testing to see what I can and cannot do. I now realize that I had got the balance between work and pleasure and family life wrong. I used to work an awful lot – more than I needed to probably. I'm trying to remedy that and looking forward to more leisure.'

Anyone returning to work should be prepared for some very mixed reactions from colleagues – rather similar to those you have encountered from friends and family. Some of them will be too embarrassed to mention your illness, unless you mention it first, and if you do not meet them half way you may find their apparent lack of concern rather hurtful.

APPLYING FOR JOBS

Sometimes, because you have lost your previous job, or you need a change, you will need to apply for a new job. In theory, there is no need to volunteer the fact that you have been treated for cancer. However, if you took a lengthy period off work, you will need to consider how to fill any gaps in your curriculum vitae. One way of overcoming this is to organize the information according to your various skills and experience, rather than in date order.

You should assume that any gap in your work record will be

noticed and be ready for questions like, 'Why did you leave your last job?', or, 'Why did you miss work for six months?' Have a truthful but very positive answer prepared that emphasizes your ability to do the job for which you have applied. For instance, you might say that you were successfully treated for cancer X, and that you are now in excellent health, and have no disabilities that would interfere with your ability to do the job.

If you are presented with a form asking you to fill in your medical history, you must give honest answers to questions like 'Have you had surgery in the past year?' or 'Specify any serious illness for which you have been treated in the past five years.' If you lie and the lie is found out, your employer has grounds to dismiss you.

However, it is unwise simply to fill in forms with answers like 'yes' and 'bowel cancer'. Use another sheet of paper, if necessary to amplify your answer, emphasizing your current good health, ability to do the job, and anything positive you may have been told about your prognosis. It will be necessary to sell your good health in the way you sell your other abilities. And, of course, if you are still feeling vulnerable, this can be easier said than done.

Sharon returned to her old job two months after treatment for cervical cancer, but then wanted to make a change. 'People told me the only way I would get a job was to tell lies on the health forms. I didn't listen, because I knew I didn't want to start a new job with a lie. I filled in a lot of forms, and didn't get interviews. I also had three interviews where people skirted round my cancer, and I felt it was certainly a factor in their decision not to employ me. In the end I was taken on by an organization that had offered me a job before I developed cancer. Even so, they were very dubious, and insisted I took a medical.'

Many people need more than the two months sick leave that Sharon allowed herself, and often a gradual return to work is recommended.

Samantha, diagnosed with breast cancer at 24, found it difficult to return to her supermarket job. She explained: 'My boss had said he would hold my job open for me, but when I went back I found that he expected me to work one long day. I really needed to build up with a few hours a day. I just couldn't do nine hours at a stretch, so I went back on the sick for a few more weeks. My boss couldn't understand it and accused me of being a scrounger.'

Several months later, after building up her confidence with

part-time work, Samantha began to apply for full-time jobs. She said: 'One interview came to a halt when they found out about the breast cancer, and when I applied for other jobs I heard nothing more after filling in the forms. I was beginning to think I would never work again, when I was offered a job with the local supermarket. Afterwards, I found out that two other girls who'd been treated for breast cancer also worked there. Getting dressed in the morning and going to work just like anyone else was absolutely great.'

BENEFITS

Sickness benefits systems can be complex, and it is easy to miss out on your entitlement. For employees in the UK, Statutory Sick Pay currently lasts for up to 28 weeks. If you are still ill after this time, then you may automatically qualify for Incapacity Benefit paid at the lower rate for up to 28 weeks. After 28 weeks, short-term Incapacity Benefit is paid at a slightly higher rate, and if you are still sick after a year, you qualify for the long-term rate. People who are terminally ill may be able to get short-term Incapacity Benefit at the long-term rate after they have been sick for 28 weeks.

Incapacity Benefit is not affected by any savings you or your partner may have, nor by any occupational pension or sick pay you may get, although you may need to pay income tax on your benefit.

To top up a low income, whether from benefits or part-time work, you can claim Income Support. The amount depends on your circumstances and the level of any income or savings of you and your partner. Income Support can help with mortgage interest payments.

You cannot generally get Income Support if you have a partner who works for 16 hours a week or more, but you may still be entitled to Housing Benefit or Council Tax Benefit to help with rent or council tax payments.

If you need help with personal care or you have mobility difficulties, you may be entitled to Disability Living Allowance. This benefit is tax-free, is not affected by your income or savings and you do not need to have paid any National Insurance contributions to qualify for it.

Benefits and entitlement rules change quite often, so it is worth contacting the Citizens Advice Bureau or a local advice agency to make sure you are not missing out. The DSS Benefits

Agency (see page 148) runs a freeline phone service where you can enquire about your own entitlement. The call is confidential and nothing you ask or say will go on your file. If you find it difficult to get a reply to your question during office hours, try between 7 p.m. and 8 p.m., when the lines may be quieter.

Some people would like to return to work, but fear losing their benefits and then finding they can't cope full-time. In fact, there are various benefits that allow you to gradually build up your hours without being out of pocket. These include the therapeutic earnings rule, where a letter from your doctor is needed, and you must work less than 16 hours a week, and the Disability Working Allowance.

If you do go back to work full-time or part-time, and realize within a few weeks that you have made a mistake, you can usually go back on benefit. For this reason it is worth reviewing how you are coping once you have been off benefit for four or five weeks. At the time of writing, it was more difficult to return to benefits if you had been back at work for more than eight weeks.

The Disability Alliance has a benefits helpline, and its annual publication, the *Disability Rights Handbook*, has a lot of information that is relevant to people with cancer. The charity CancerLink has a useful booklet on Cancer and Employment or, again, you can consult the DSS free phone line.

If you live in the US, the American Cancer Society can help you find local agencies that respond to problems over employment and insurance rights.

MAKING A WILL

For the cancer patient, making a will is not a sign that you are 'giving up' and is really something which everyone should do. Even if we cannot control the timing and manner of our dying, the making of a will helps to restore some control over what happens afterwards. It should also reduce some of the distress faced by our families. If you make your wishes absolutely clear, at a time when you are fit and well, it is difficult for those who are left behind to squabble or claim that you were unduly influenced. (And regrettably such disputes often arise when wills are made towards the end of a final illness.)

Many people feel more secure about a will drawn up by a solicitor (attorney). In the US, in particular, a lawyer-drawn will is less likely to be challenged. If you decide to write your own will, a number of charities including BACUP have leaflets, advising you on how to proceed. Will forms can be purchased from major stationers.

LIVING WILLS

Now recognized in a number of countries, living wills have nothing to do with our worldly goods. These documents make it clear that you do not want your life prolonged by medical intervention if your condition is hopeless, and you have no reasonable chance of recovery. Although any patient can refuse medical treatment at any time, the living will covers the eventuality that you will be so ill (or unconscious) that you are unable to make your wishes clear.

Make copies of your living will for your family doctor (and possibly specialist) to add to your medical records, and also for close relatives, and leave the document with your other personal papers. Unfortunately, the pain of bereavement is often expressed in the form of bitter quarrelling among relatives who are left: making your views clear in a dated document when you are well and have all your mental faculties will help to avoid this unnecessary grief.

In the UK, living wills are available from the Voluntary Euthanasia Society (see page 149). In the US, each state has its own laws concerning living wills and power of attorney. These should be widely available in local hospitals, law libraries and attorneys' offices. Otherwise the Cancer Information Service (see page 150) can advise on how to obtain this information.

FINDING THE BEST MEDICAL CARE

It would be wonderful to write that anyone living anywhere will have access to the best cancer treatment available. Unfortunately, it would not be true. If you need further treatment, you may be lucky enough to live near a specialist centre that is providing state-of-the-art treatment. However, it is equally likely that you will not be so fortunate, and that you will need to be vigilant to ensure you get the best out of the health system at this important point in your life.

THE ROLE OF THE FAMILY DOCTOR

The cancer charities say that many people are unable to work the NHS effectively, because they do not understand how the system operates. Your family doctor acts as the gatekeeper to the NHS, opening doors so that you can see the right consultant, and indicating to that consultant the urgency of your case. As most patients spend only a short time in hospital before returning to their normal lives, the hospital should keep your family doctor informed about its clinical findings, and any treatment you have received, so that he or she can continue your care.

If, after your treatment has been completed, you realize you do not fully understand what has happened, or the implications, you should see your family doctor. He or she should either be able to answer your questions or refer you back to the hospital. If you need psychological help, physiotherapy or the services of a pain specialist, it is your family doctor who will open the door.

To help you effectively, your family doctor needs to be familiar with your local cancer services, and prepared to argue your case with the funding authorities if necessary. He or she will need to be interested enough to offer you continuing support in the months that follow your treatment. This is a partnership, and it is reasonable to expect that you confide in your family doctor. This means telling him or her when you are unable to follow medical advice (perhaps because the suggested treatment is making you ill), and of any other therapies you are trying.

An open-minded family doctor should welcome any complementary therapy that makes you feel better, and that does not interfere with your physical health. If you are not happy with your family doctor – or simply find you don't get on together – you can go to another doctor's practice and ask to be registered. You do not have to tell your doctor why you want to change practices.

FINDING THE RIGHT HOSPITAL

If you need further medical care, you may be pleasantly surprised by the changes you encounter. Thanks to the work of pressure groups, cancer charities and patient advocacy groups, there is a gradual switch to caring for the welfare of the whole person, rather than simply the diseased part.

Busy hospital staff do not always remember to tell you about the full range of services that are available, so watch the notice boards, look out for leaflets, and, of course – ask! In some cases, you may be presenting such a calm front that it simply does not occur to anyone that you might need counselling, or feel you would like to try a support group.

Although the US offers excellent medical care, patients have the additional hurdle of having to ensure their health insurance policies will cover the cost. This is a very complex issue, and if your cover is inadequate, you really need personal, rather than general, advice. The American Cancer Society emphasizes the importance of letting your doctor know as soon as you encounter any insurance difficulties.

It is tempting to put the 'nasty' letter from the insurance company aside, especially if you are already feeling rather low. Shelving the problem will not help you forget it, so get help quickly. Your hospital's social service office should be able to assist, and to direct you to other sources of help. Often, even for patients who are inadequately insured, it is possible to ensure continuity of treatment. This is a problem that frequently crops up and you need to enlist the help of agencies who are experts in dealing with it – fast. Other sources of help include social workers and your local office of the American Cancer Society.

In the UK, the government has now recognized that cancer patients have a right to the care of a specialist, although as yet that intention had not yet been translated into action. Patient power is forcing many doctors to evaluate the way they practise, and to decide whether they want to specialize in cancer treatment, or pass patients on to others who have chosen to do so. However, you may find that getting the best possible medical care for yourself involves some personal effort – and perhaps even some campaigning.

Becky Miles was diagnosed with advanced Hodgkins Disease in 1990. After being referred to her ninth doctor in nine months she realized she was not getting the expert help she needed to save her life. She explains: 'Neither my GP nor the cancer help lines seemed able to help me find the doctor I needed. It was only because I had medical friends that I was able to work the system.'

Once Becky's treatment was successfully completed, she set up the National Cancer Alliance, which is committed to ensuring improvements in cancer treatment and care are made quickly. Becky explains: 'Cancer patients often need a combination of treatments – surgery, drugs, radiotherapy, dietary advice and counselling to name just a few. It seems absurdly simple to expect such patients to have access to specialists working in a multidisciplinary team. But for many people it just isn't happening.'

The UK is fortunate compared with many other countries in having a health service that is comprehensive and free of charge. Unfortunately for cancer patients, this comprehensive cover can be spread very thinly. For instance, in East Anglia, in 1995, there was a cancer centre for every 700,000 of the population. In the North West region, there was a centre for every 3,200,000 of the population. In fact, the UK had fewer cancer specialists per head of population than any other European country apart from Portugal.

You may wonder if this really matters, provided you get the right treatment at the right time. Research has shown that, as we might expect, specialists tend to get better results. Despite this, fewer than 50 per cent of cancer patients were seen by a specialist in 1995. The government is now attempting to remedy the situation by setting up cancer units in district hospitals, which will be led by a cancer specialist. These should provide surgery, radiotherapy and drug treatments on the same site and be capable of dealing with the commonest cancers, e.g. breast, bowel and lung.

When more specialized treatment is required than the units are able to offer (or where children and adolescents are involved), patients will be referred to designated cancer centres. So how do you judge whether you are being treated in the right place?

Dr Maurice Slevin, says: 'I would advise patients to go to a centre where they know research is being carried out. In research centres, the treatments will be up to date, and will have been agreed by a panel of specialists. Doctors who are involved in research practise at a higher level. Hospitals that are satellites of specialist centres are fine – because they will be following the same guidelines.' If you want to find out if your cancer unit is involved in research, and your family doctor cannot tell you, then you should try the BACUP information line.

Being seen by the 'top' specialist in your disease does not solve all your treatment problems. Highly regarded specialists can have very long lists of patients, frequent international lecture commitments and are likely to spend their precious time with the most complex 'cases'. If your professor or consultant is heading a competent and well-briefed team of doctors, this problem can easily be mitigated. Even so, you will be lucky if your doctor has time to deal with all your concerns about your cancer.

Or you may have the reverse problem. Your doctor is all too eager to give you lots of technical information, but you find that you simply can't take it in. This does not mean you are stupid. Everyone finds it hard to absorb more than a limited amount of new facts, even when the subject is not as important as their future health. It is quite likely that you will still be trying to remember whether you should be taking the pink pills every other day while the specialist is telling you something important about side effects. This is where the tape recorder (or friend with a notebook) can come into their own.

If you are unhappy with the advice you have been given, or think that your consultant has written you off, you have the right to ask for (although not to get) a second opinion. If you are prepared to see another specialist at the same hospital, your consultant should be able to arrange this (provided there is another specialist in the same field). Otherwise you will have to go back and ask your family doctor to arrange this. Most people recognize the importance of decisions about cancer treatment and will not lightly refuse such a request.

It may be that you are perfectly happy with the treatment you've received, but feel that you want to go back to see the consultant to discuss a new concern. If so, it is worth ringing the unit and speaking directly to the consultant's secretary. This will sometimes open the door for you, but as the NHS becomes more bureaucratic you may find that you have to go back to the gatekeeper, your family doctor. If you are involved in research (see the section on clinical trials, page 90), you may find that the research nurse attached to the project is a helpful source of further information – or can tell you where to find out what you need to know.

If you feel that your hospital specialist does not specialize in your particular type of cancer, you may need to undertake some research. The National Cancer Alliance has now produced a directory that identifies cancer specialists geographically, and by their areas of interest. Unfortunately, cancer surgeons have not yet worked out their accreditation system, and so are not included in the directory. Inclusion does not, in any case, count as an endorsement, but having a specialist's name has to be better than not having a name.

The BACUP helpline, although similarly unable to endorse any particular doctor, should be able to help you locate specialists in your particular type of cancer. The cancer charities can also sometimes help, as they fund research into many types of cancer treatment.

KEEPING CONTROL OVER HEALTH DECISIONS

Your local hospital is dealing with hundreds of patients every week, and it is unsafe to expect the organization to be foolproof. Margaret queried the fact that at 52 she had not been called up for the national breast-screening programme. Her family doctor offered to arrange a mammogram 'if you are worried', but in fact she was invited for screening two weeks later. When the breast x-ray proved to be abnormal, Margaret was called to the screening centre, where two doctors started to argue over whether her breast lump needed to be treated.

Margaret said: 'The woman doctor in charge said she wanted to see me in six months time, but I could see that the other doctor and the nurse who took the x-ray were very unhappy about this. I went back to my family doctor, who sent me to see a specialist. The specialist examined me and said immediately that the lump was malignant. He was very angry with the woman doctor for not sending me to see him, and said it was lucky I had insisted on a second opinion. But it wasn't luck. I don't think you can leave something as important as this to chance – especially when the doctors themselves were disagreeing.'

Fifteen years before her breast cancer was diagnosed, Margaret was found to have stomach cancer. She still needs regular gastroscopies (examinations of her oesophagus and duodenum) to check the disease has not returned. She said: 'I keep an eye on the calendar, and if the appointment doesn't come through when I expect it, I ring up – not to complain, but just to make sure. I know how many people they deal with and how easy it is to slip through the net.'

DIFFICULT TREATMENT DECISIONS

When you are first diagnosed with cancer, the situation is fairly clear: you want the disease treated as vigorously as possible, in the hope of a cure. This may continue to be the case if you have a first or second recurrence of your cancer. For many people cancer is a chronic condition: they remain well for most of the time, but periodically need to 'zap' it with a new treatment.

However, the time may come when your treatment options are much less clear cut, and when your doctors themselves seem uncertain as to whether or not you will benefit from further curative therapy. Alternatively, in the hope of buying some more time, they may offer you a treatment that you know has unpleasant side effects and you may no longer be prepared to tolerate them.

Another dilemma occurs when your doctors seem to want to give up on you, when you are not ready to give up yourself, and want to try any treatment, no matter how remote the chances of success. Your family and friends may also have an input here. You may feel that they are not ready to lose you, or cannot manage without you. Conversely, you may feel that they have had enough of the pain of caring for you.

All this can make your decision very hard, and you may need to go back to first principles. It is your life, and no one else's. No matter how close you are to your family and friends, they cannot know exactly how you feel (because you will have often shielded them from your true feelings). This is one time when you have to work to your own agenda, and no one else's.

The important thing to remember is that you can change your mind at any stage. You can refuse to continue with a treatment once you have started it, or you can change your mind about a therapy that you had initially refused.

Stopping treatment will not mean your doctor ceases to care for you, and when you stop talking about cures, you should start talking about palliative therapies that will relieve your symptoms and improve your quality of life.

If you disagree with the decision to stop active treatment, you should ask for a second opinion. You may also want to enquire if you may qualify for entry into a clinical trial of a new treatment into your condition.

AGEISM

Unfortunately, there is some evidence that older patients are under-treated because doctors believe they are sparing them from distress. In fact, new research from the UK, other European countries and the US has shown that older patients often respond better to chemotherapy, with fewer side effects, than do younger people. Your treatment should be given on the basis of your physical condition at the time, and the nature and stage of your cancer. If you suspect that you are being discriminated against because of age (even with the best possible intentions), then you may need to question the decision and, if necessary, ask for a second opinion.

CLINICAL TRIALS

One of the most common queries made to the cancer charities comes from patients whose doctors say that no more curative therapies are available. Often (although not always) there is clinical research going on somewhere in the country that might be relevant to such patients. However, there is no guarantee that inclusion in such a trial will lengthen your life, or indeed that you will be accepted as a participant. New cancer drugs and different treatment regimes are generally tried first on patients for whom other treatments have failed. If you feel that any avenue is worth exploring, you will need to start making some enquiries.

For patients in the US, it could hardly be easier. They simply have to call the Cancer Information Service (see page 150), which can immediately provide the information they need from the Physician Data Query system (PDQ). This lists the latest treatments, research studies and clinical trials.

Unfortunately, no single body yet holds this information in the UK, although it is worth contacting the Imperial Cancer Research Fund or the Cancer Research Campaign, or any charity with an interest in your type of cancer. Eventually the British hope to imitate the PDQ system.

Trying a new treatment offers only a thin hope of success, but if you decide to go down this road, do not feel that you are asking for favours. Doctors frequently find it difficult to recruit enough patients for a particular trial from their own 'patch'. Their reputations (and promotions) are partly built on successful research studies. If you are eligible, i.e. you are the kind of patient needed for this particular piece of research, then you are furthering medical knowledge in the hope of buying more time – a fair trade for all concerned.

The very first human test of a brand-new treatment, known as a phase I trial, aims to establish the correct dose in order to achieve the maximum cancer-killing effect with the minimum side effects. These trials involve small numbers of people who start with low doses that are gradually increased. If all your other options have been exhausted, you may be prepared to take part in this type of research. In doing so, you are more likely to help other patients than yourself, although phase I trials do very occasionally produce results that seem almost miraculous in people for whom all other treatments have failed.

In a phase II trial, further information is gathered about the correct dose, and the drug is often tested on several types of cancer. Both phase I and phase II trials generally involve no more than a couple of dozen participants – and there is no doubt that they do very occasionally buy extra years of life for people whose future was being measured by the week.

When Danny was 23, he was gravely ill with testicular teratoma and expected to live only a few more weeks. As a last resort, he was treated with a new, experimental drug combination that included the platinum-based drug, cisplatin. It later became a standard therapy, saving thousands of young men all over the world from what had once been a killer disease.

Seventeen years later Danny was still alive and well. He said: 'The cancer was in my lymph nodes and had spread all over my body. My wife and mother were told I would be dead within weeks. Then a different doctor came along and gave me some new drugs. He told me I was a guinea pig. The side effects were awful, but I think they have refined the treatment since. And it saved my life.'

A hospice place had been found for Margaret, 37, when doctors decided that surgery alone would not cure her stomach cancer. Her husband was told she was unlikely to survive for three months. After removing two thirds of her stomach, Margaret's doctor decided to try chemotherapy, although it had no track record with Margaret's type of cancer.

Seventeen years later, Margaret commented: 'I thought I would never see my children grow up, and now I've got grandchildren. The chemotherapy went on for two and a half years. I got used to the idea that I would carry on with the housework while being sick at the beginning of the week, and work part-time at the end of the week. They kept saying it would stop after six months, and then I had another six months, and then another. There's no doubt in my mind that it saved me. There was a group of us with the same cancer, and I'm told I was the only survivor. The professor used to show me off and describe me as his star lady. The others who had been diagnosed at the same time as me had all died.'

You do not have to have exhausted conventional treatment to be enrolled into a clinical trial, however. Many cancer patients are asked to take part in research in which one treatment is being compared with another – a phase III trial involving hundreds and sometimes thousands of patients.

The objective may be to establish whether a particular dose of a drug works better than a slightly higher or lower dose, or whether that drug works better in combination with another, or to compare a new treatment with an established one.

Trials do not only compare drugs, but also cover surgical procedures, radiotherapy and psychological therapies. At the same time, parallel studies may be carried out to measure the effects of treatment on your quality of life.

This type of research is randomized, which means that a computer allocates you at random to one of the treatments being compared. When possible it is also 'double blind' which means that neither you, nor your doctor, know which treatment you are on. Clinical trials should be carefully monitored by hospital ethics committees. They may involve patients from other hospitals in your home country and abroad. They are carried out to try to define the best possible treatment for each type of cancer.

No one can force you to take part in a trial, and you can drop out at any stage. However, patients who take part in trials tend to be more carefully monitored and to do better than those who are not – almost regardless of the treatment which is being tested.

If you are not benefiting from the trial treatment, your doctor will withdraw you from the study and try something else (if this is appropriate). Entering a trial may involve you in an increased number of hospital visits and more blood tests and other checks of your general health. These are to safeguard you from possible problems associated with the new treatment.

Every so often doctors will break the code and analyse the results for a subset of patients. If one treatment turns out to be far superior to the others, the trial will be stopped and everyone will be switched to the better treatment. Otherwise the trial will continue to its planned endpoint, which may be as long as five or ten years.

CHAPTER 8

EFFECTIVE
SELF-HELP

For months I'd been depressed without a cause
Restless, lethargic, given to tears behind closed doors,
Seeing the bad in every situation – hating myself.
At last I had a cause, and all my strengths renewed,
I fought my way through tests and scans
Informing relatives, making a will,
And freezing down as much as I could cook.

SHARON WILLMOTT

REGAINING CONTROL

There is a lot of argument about what is the 'correct' mental attitude for the cancer patient who wants to survive. This can be infuriating if you have cancer. You probably prefer not to see yourself as a patient at all, but as someone who has been successfully treated for a serious medical condition. You may think it is presumptuous for anyone who has not had cancer to tell you what you should be thinking and feeling.

If you are symptom-free, it should not matter whether your illness was cancer or influenza: you are now a well person. But, as you have discovered, it doesn't work like that. Anyone who has had cancer is labelled by the media as a 'cancer victim'. People who survive heart attacks are not similarly labelled, although their future is arguably even more uncertain.

Cancer patients often feel that they have lost control of their personal situations, and have become public property not only of the doctors, but also of their friends and relatives who discuss their 'case'. 'I felt that in 24 hours, in the eyes of the world, I had changed into an entirely different person,' says Debbie, describing the period when her breast cancer was diagnosed.

'One of the worst parts was the feeling that I had lost the sense of ownership of my body, it was as if the world was happening outside me. Yet when, after nine months, my treatment stopped, I felt as if I had been cast adrift.'

Samantha, who also had breast cancer, said: 'At the time of my treatment, I didn't feel as if my life belonged to me. Everyone else seemed to be making the important decisions.'

MIND OVER BODY?

People who have been treated for cancer are often told by well-meaning friends that they must 'think positive'. Such patronizing advice is on a par with 'pull yourself together'. If it were that easy, there would be no need to utter the exhortation.

So what are the facts about mental attitude? Research has shown that people who exhibit a lot of emotional distress during cancer treatment can benefit from psychotherapy. This helps them adopt a more positive attitude to their futures, and enhances their quality of life. The medical profession is sufficiently convinced of the value of such supportive therapy to allow psychologists and psychotherapists to join the cancer team. Some research suggests that people with positive attitudes to their disease survive for longer than those who feel hopeless or resigned to their fate. Other studies have found no such effect. In short, the evidence is contradictory.

If you read a statement which is categorical about the effectiveness of mental attitude on survival (or, indeed, its ineffectiveness) then you should smell a rat. The author is probably demonstrating publication bias. This occurs when people who want to make a case simply cite the research studies which support them, and ignore all the others.

So where does this leave you? Common sense suggests that a strong, positive approach to life will not be enough to overwhelm an advanced cancer that has spread throughout the body. Otherwise the 'nice guys' or feisty, positive thinkers like John Wayne would go on forever.

Dr Harold H. Benjamin was founder of the Wellness Community in Santa Monica, California, and a firm believer in positive thinking. In his book, *From Victim to Victor*, he wrote:

'We have always known there is no such thing as a sure cure. Promises that "if you do what we tell you, then you will get well" are not messages of false hope; they're either fraud or stupidity... Just as life does not end with the diagnosis of cancer, life does not end when the possibility of recovery becomes remote. Life goes on as long as life goes on.'

Prof. Karol Sikora, a leading cancer physician, and Deputy Director of the Imperial Cancer Research Fund, broadly agrees. He said: 'I certainly believe in the relationship between the mind and the body when it comes to cancer treatment. When people have a positive approach they cope better with their disease, and also with the treatment. And if they tolerate the treatment better, they are more likely to respond.

'On many occasions, I have been surprised by patients who have survived for much longer than anyone would have expected. Sometimes they have been keeping themselves going for family celebrations – sometimes there is no obvious reason why they do so well. Having said all that, some tumours are so aggressive that no matter how positive you are, it will make no difference to your survival.'

Nevertheless, cancer is a process, and it seems logical that some people will have disease that is at a borderline stage where it could either be destroyed or progress. At that point, it seems fair to argue that a strong mental attitude could tip the balance in your favour. Cancer cells are not only killed by medical treatments, but also by your own immune system, which can overwhelm small numbers of 'foreign invaders'.

Stress researchers suggest that we have a limited amount of energy to spend on physical and mental trauma. If we use too much of it to adapt to our emotional distress, we may end up lacking the reserves we need to fight off a serious challenge to our physical health. At the very least, negative emotions such as fear and depression are likely to make you feel ill and complicate your recovery.

Discovering that you have the ability to reduce your stress, and improve the way you feel about life, helps restore some personal control. It could even be a life saver. But can people change their mental attitudes?

Research suggests that they can – provided they wish to do so. No psychiatrist or doctor can help a patient who does not want to get well. But truly negative people would not be reading this book, because they would have convinced themselves that nothing they could do would make a difference. If you think you can change, then you can.

THE MAINSTREAM MEDICAL VIEW

So what do doctors regard as the ideal survivor's mentality? Dr Maurice Slevin says: 'Some of the most successful copers are people who are able to forget about their cancers for much of the time. They may acknowledge that there is a high risk of recurrence, but they will say firmly, I am choosing not to think about it. They tell me that whatever I say about their prognosis, they have decided they are going to do well, and their cancer is going to stay away. Sometimes they ask me what I think is going to happen, and when I tell them my opinion, will comment, "It is not going to happen to me."

'The ones who do less well are overwhelmed by their cancer and won't even plan for next week, let alone think about going away on holiday.'

Jim, whose doctor told him his oesophageal cancer was incurable, said: 'When I go for check-ups, my doctor is surprised by how well I look. In fact, he says I look better than he does.' Jim is continuing to plant his garden and run his business, and at 68 he regards neither his age nor his cancer as reasons to retire.

Dr Amanda Ramirez says: 'The people who do best psychologically have a realistic awareness of their prognosis, but find some way of putting it on the back burner. In everyday life, they don't think about cancer very often.

'Some people achieve this when they go back to work, although I worry about those who go back too early before they have had time to air all their concerns, sort out their feelings, and then put the subject of cancer to the back of their minds.

'It is normal and psychologically healthy to have sad moments when you acknowledge that the cancer may come back. People who cope well will find ways of making sure they do not dwell on these thoughts for too long.'

Another strategy that helps patients cope better is the ability to derive some benefit from the experience of having cancer. These people are just as upset over their illness at the time of diagnosis as everyone else, and are just as worried about their futures. However, they are able to see some positive gains in the experience, such as becoming closer to their families, becoming less concerned with trivia and minor setbacks in life, and gaining a better appreciation of natural beauty and the changing seasons.

The people who cope least well are those with a lot of other worries on their plates, in addition to their cancers. These vulnerable individuals are particularly likely to need psychological support, and will need to find ways of becoming more selfish, and to make sure the burden of family and financial worry is spread more fairly.

Danny was treated for testicular teratoma 17 years ago, and had a local recurrence three years ago. He said: 'I have a fatalistic approach to my cancer. There are certain things you can do to try to keep it at bay, such as avoiding smoking and keeping fit. I'm a vegetarian for health reasons. But at the end of the day, whether or not my cancer comes back is out of my hands. You have to go with the flow.'

Sharon would be the first to admit that her approach to her cervical cancer verged on the obsessive, as she filled her day with a programme of mental and physical exercise to combat cancer. She is also proof that a negative mental attitude is not an immediate kiss of death. She said: 'The consultant had been very pessimistic and for the first few months, I was preparing myself for death. I was aiming to dissolve my personality and merge into the great nothing – all I wanted to do was become serene and luminous and fade out. Newspapers and TV news were irrelevant to me.'

However, Sharon's newly acquired calm was shattered when she thought, wrongly, that her cancer had recurred. Once this false alarm was resolved she continued with what she described as her 'rather rarefied existence'.

She found talking freely about her cancer, to anyone who would listen, helped sort out her true feelings. She said: 'I suppose it was like grieving, when you talk about something you have lost in an attempt to get rid of the sadness. After about six months, I realized my disease had not recurred and I would have to return to life in the here and now.'

Gradually Sharon was able to forget her cancer for an hour, then half a day, and then she realized she had gone a whole day without thinking about it. 'Finally, after about two years, I realized I could meet new people without needing to tell them about my cancer. It just wasn't relevant any more.'

THE COMPLEMENTARY THERAPIST'S VIEW

Dr Rosy Daniels says: 'Doctors tend to treat cancer as if it is an inexorable process, and as if nothing you can do can make any difference. It is a big message and you need to wipe it out of your psyche. The nurturing and self-healing part of medicine is left out of the picture, and yet it is very potent.

'If you are fearful, but are told there is nothing you can do about your illness, then all the energy you might have used for self-help gets cycled back into fear. When our spirits are crushed, our ability to fight illness is crushed, no matter what vitamins and drugs we put into our bodies.

'You need to dare to imagine that you can be whole and well and strong again. So often, after people are given their diagnosis, they stop visualizing themselves on holiday, or enjoying things that might happen in the future.'

Dr Daniels describes three stages by which psychological health is regained. Firstly, when people are at their lowest ebb, she suggests a visit to a healer. After this, she recommends relaxation, where the body shifts into a nurturing stage – 'something cats and dogs do naturally'. The third therapy is meditation, where the mind is allowed to become still. 'People have been healed by meditation alone,' she says.

One of the most important objectives of Bristol Cancer Help Centre is to restore hope to people who feel their cases are hopeless. There is, after all, no form of cancer that does not have some survivors. Many of the Bristol therapies help relieve stress and restore inner calm and a sense of personal control, so that the body can heal itself. 'We have seen people come back from the edge of death and get well and strong again. Everything is possible,' concludes Dr Daniels.

COMING TO TERMS WITH YOUR SITUATION

Positive attitudes do not just descend on you overnight. If you want to muster your psychological resources to do battle against your cancer, you will need to learn to recognize negative thoughts and attitudes, challenge them, and turn them around (see Chapter 2, page 20).

Do not be too hard on yourself, however. Everyone, regardless of whether they have cancer, occasionally feels sad at the thought of their own death and wonders how the family will cope. Cancer makes the possibility of death more real, and dealing with those feelings is part of your acceptance of the situation.

You will need to recognize when other people (including the medical profession) are bringing you down to their own level of pessimism, because this can be a threat to your emotional well-being. The decision over whether to ignore them, or try to persuade them that their attitudes are unhelpful and unfounded, is up to you. Some previously mild-mannered people are surprised by the freedom a life-threatening diagnosis gives them to express their real feelings and needs.

Jeanette's brain tumour is benign, but the term is rather a misnomer. It is in the base of her brain, and if it grows any larger, there is no guarantee that a future operation will be successful. She said: 'For as long as I can remember, I have avoided confrontations with people. I had always really wanted to work in a shop, but I didn't think I could be spared from the business that my husband and I run together. When I recovered from my treatment, I decided to work in a charity shop. I enjoyed it, and I found the business has survived perfectly well without me being there every day.'

Sylvia, who was treated for cervical cancer, said: 'Although my five children had grown up, I used to hesitate to go away in case they needed me to baby-sit their children. I still baby-sit, but I don't let people take me for granted any more. They used to come to me for Sunday dinner, but now they take turns to cook for me.'

Having turned round your thinking, you then need to think about the psychological weak spots that might be delaying your recovery.

FACTORS THAT CAN DELAY RECOVERY

- Self-blame and poor self-image
- Inability to 'make sense' of what has happened
- Overwhelming stress
- Long-standing anger and resentment
- Fear of recurrence/inability to plan ahead

SELF-IMAGE

One of the most frightening things about cancer is its random nature. Not surprisingly many people prefer to blame themselves or some outside force for their illness, rather than accept that it simply happened. Self-blame (and indeed the blame of others) knocks you off your recovery path and straight into a cul-de-sac.

Most cancers are not fully explicable, or carry explanations such as genetic susceptibility that take you no further. The thought that you caused your own cancer, e.g. by smoking, carries a particular bitterness. Your pain and distress are just as bad as anyone else's, and yet you feel that others are thinking that you brought it on yourself.

Your first step has to be to forgive yourself – perhaps by imagining a friend in the same situation. You would not accuse your friend of deliberately giving himself cancer, because no sane person would do that. You might argue, in your friend's defence, that he was hooked on his cigarettes, and despite numerous attempts had failed to quit. You might also add that many people smoke without developing cancer. Yes, your actions would be different if you could turn back the clock, but that is impossible. But while you cannot change the past, you can have a say in what you will do in the future.

Some people find it helpful to concentrate on simple statements – positive affirmations – of how they feel about their situation. You might try the following, or consider drawing up your own statement:

- Regardless of how I react to my situation, my feelings are my own, and they are perfectly valid
- I deserve to be treated with respect and dignity, and I respect myself
- Whatever happens to my body, I will always remain at peace with myself

Complications following radiotherapy meant that Sylvia hardly dared stray far from a lavatory. A colostomy operation liberated her, but at first she felt self-conscious and fearful that people could somehow tell she was different.

Sylvia said: 'One day, I realized I couldn't just curl up feeling sorry for myself. I now make a point of dressing myself up whenever I go out – far more than I did before I was ill. I put on make-up, nice clothes, and I get my hair done. I wear skirts again, and I feel good about myself.'

Sally, an ex-dancer who was also treated for cervical cancer, was determined from the outset that cancer would not change the way she felt about herself. She did not need a colostomy, but the swelling of her legs, caused by lymphoedema, provide a constant reminder that she has been treated for cancer.

Sally says: 'I'd never looked on myself as a victim or a likely cancer patient – it was not the way I saw myself dying. I thought that they'd picked the wrong person here. I was told I had a fifty-fifty chance of survival.

'I do have bad days, everyone does, but you have to see them as a hiccup and not a sign you're a negative person. No one can be positive all the time, but I try to be ready for the black moments. I don't think there's any point in sloping around, looking less than my usual self. When I am low, I put on my best shoes, and my favourite lipstick and lots of scent. It's my theatrical background coming out, I think – the feeling the show must go on.'

MAKING SENSE OF YOUR CANCER

In her book, *Time on Our Side*, psychologist Dorothy Rowe explains the futility of trying to make sense out of what is essentially senseless. She says many people like to think they live in a Just World. Yet, in fact, it is essential for our psychological survival to recognize that there is no natural justice, and that we live in a real world, where anything can and does happen.

Dr Rowe writes: 'Coming to terms is an awareness that everything changes and that is all right. . . . It is accepting that we have suffered wounds and losses for which there is no recompense. There was no special reason why we suffered. We were simply unlucky to have been in that particular place at that particular time. However, being unlucky in the past does not mean that we won't be lucky in the future. . . .

'Part of coming to terms is accepting the presence of death in our lives, and recognizing its importance. This means recognizing that everyone will die and that there are no exceptions, recognizing that the process cannot be prettified or glossed over no matter how we might try, and recognizing how death can show us what is important in our lives.'

If you have strong religious beliefs, you may not accept Dr Rowe's analysis. The belief that your illness is part of God's plan or that you are being protected by a greater being can be immensely comforting, as is the acceptance that all of life and death is natural. If you feel that that your illness occurred because God is punishing you, then you should discuss those views with a minister or priest from your church. Such views are likely to be erroneous.

Jim, 68, whose doctors have given him little hope of a cure, said: 'I have always believed there is something out there which is greater than mankind, and I am in no doubt that this power can help me through this problem.'

Jane, 51, says her experience of breast cancer five years ago has intensified her religious faith. 'Before I got cancer, I was terrified of getting it. Now, I feel glad that I've had cancer, because it has helped prove God to me. I thought nothing could take my fear away, and then God did.'

OVERCOMING STRESS

It is clearly nonsense to regard stress as a twentieth-century plague. Ever since we came down from the trees, men and women have had to worry about the very real possibility of starving or freezing to death, or being killed by a human or animal predator. A regular food supply, warmth and shelter have seldom been guaranteed.

Stress helps us to catch trains on time, finish a task and agree to take on new work. It brings challenge and variety into our lives. It accompanies family arguments, bereavements, job changes and the sudden, unpredictable breakdown of the washing machine and car. Without stress no one would ever marry or have children, or change jobs, or move house. Stress only damages our health when it is perceived as distressing.

You can partially insulate yourself from unwarranted distress by accepting changes and misfortunes as part of normal life, and refusing to use the 'S' word. However, when stress becomes unmanageable, you need to pick up the warning signs and do something about it. Stress symptoms, such as headache, sleeplessness, insomnia, back pain and digestive disorders (e.g. flatulence, diarrhoea) are unpleasant, and may be mistaken for a recurrence of cancer. Stress can also intensify any pre-existing pain.

Research suggests that people who are most stress-resistant have a strong commitment to themselves, a sense of control over external events, combined with the ability to see change as a challenge rather than a threat. They accept that it is more normal for situations to change than to stay the same indefinitely.

If you are anxious and unhappy, you may feel like giving a hollow laugh at the suggestion that relaxation can solve your problems. If you could relax, you wouldn't be stressed!

However, very tense people can decide to take time for themselves and relax – and success is a potent morale booster. Simple relaxation techniques, combined with the use of your imagination to produce positive, life-enhancing images, can make a tremendous difference to the way you feel. Provided you do not expect instant results, it is possible for anyone to relax, and the techniques will undoubtedly make you feel better. Remember that relaxation does not always mean taking the phone off the hook and lying flat on the floor.

When Margaret, who has been treated for both stomach and breast cancers, wishes to unwind, she goes into her painting room. She explained: 'I paint china. I do dogs and cats, wedding plates, money boxes for children . . . you name it. I have always wanted to do something arty, and when I was first diagnosed with cancer, 18 years ago, I felt sad at the thought I'd never done it. Then, one day when I was passing an art shop, I went in on a whim and got the materials. Now I use it for enjoyment, and as a kind of therapy. There are some days when I really itch to get up into my painting room. I know it will make me feel better – it always does.'

Kevin, who was treated for testicular cancer, writes humorous articles and short stories. He says: 'My writing has become even more important to me since my diagnosis. It is a way of unwinding and of dealing with what has happened.'

Sharon uses yoga, which she says both unwinds and energizes her. More detail about relaxation techniques is given in Chapter 9 (see page 108).

DEALING WITH ANGER

Anger and resentment are perfectly legitimate feelings, provided they are not causing you harm. Martin Luther wrote: 'When I am angry, I can write, pray and preach well, for then my whole temperament is quickened, my understanding sharpened and all mundane vexations and temptations gone.'

Sometimes, however, anger can burn on for months and years. If you continue to dwell on past events, which are impossible to change, then the anger can turn inwards and become self-destructive. For instance, many of the people whose cancer experiences are described in this book had encountered long delays before diagnosis.

Jane, who had an instinct that she would develop breast cancer, had been reassured there was nothing wrong by her family doctor, well woman clinic and a private specialist whom she had paid to see. She ended up having a mastectomy, followed by a surgical implant that had to be removed following rejection problems. Although she still occasionally feels angry at the false reassurances she received, she now accepts she cannot turn back the clock.

Unfortunately, Jenny, who also had a mastectomy, thinks about her anger with her breast surgeon nearly every day of her life. He originally told Jenny she could have a breast reconstruction operation after her mastectomy, and then got an underling to tell her he had changed his mind. There is no doubt this situation was badly handled. In the end, another doctor performed the reconstruction operation, and Jenny was pleased with the result.

However, 30 months later, Jenny said: 'I'm nowhere near to putting my cancer on the back burner. On most days I still have a time when I think about the surgeon. I imagine myself telling that swine off. If I'm not doing that, I'm feeling angry with myself for not asking more questions at the time, and not being better pre-pared when they tried to tell me I couldn't have the operation.'

Jenny is bright enough to realize all this is doing her no good, but she is unable to control her thoughts.

Simon Darnley, a behavioural cognitive therapist at the Institute of Psychiatry, commented: 'It's quite common for intense anger to delay someone's recovery, whether they have a major illness, or have suffered in an accident. Most hospitals now have psychiatrists or psychologists who deal with this type of anger, and so people in this situation can get help.'

Cognitive behavioural therapy aims to get the patient to realize the consequences of their anger, and weigh up whether it is doing good or harm. Simply telling people it is harmful does not work. They have to work out the harm, and the ineffectiveness of the emotion for themselves.

If you feel anger is delaying your recovery, it may be worth considering writing down some of the questions and statements in the rest of this section – along with your responses. Do not expect to change your way of thinking in ten minutes. If you have been obsessed with a past event for many months, it may take some determined effort to rid yourself of these thoughts.

If Jenny had psychological therapy, it might take eight to 12 weeks to resolve her problem. The therapy would begin by teaching her to recognize the triggers for her anger and to question if it is reasonable always to have to experience those feelings at that particular time of day. In Jenny's case, the triggers would occur when she got dressed or showered in the morning.

Other 'homework' for Jenny would be to consider all the things she could do, no matter how outrageous, to get her own back on the surgeon. Would any of these actions achieve results, or make her feel better? How feasible were they, and what would be the consequences? Jenny would be invited to consider what the anger was doing for her, how it was helping and hindering her recovery, and what her feelings were about the surgeon.

As she set out those feelings, in speech and in writing, she would be encouraged to challenge the use of certain words and phrases. If for instance, she said, 'He has ruined my life' or, 'I'll never get over it', she would be shown how to question how closely those thoughts reflected her true situation. In Jenny's case, the doctor was only ruining her life because she thought he was.

Jenny's case is an extreme one. If you feel your anger may be hindering your recovery, and that your thoughts about what happened are running in a continuous loop, you could try a thought-stopping technique. First, you need to identify the triggers that set off your anger, and then, when you start to relive the experience, you have to say (or shout, if you are alone), 'Stop. I am not going to waste time thinking about that.'

Another technique is to draw a series of circles – the blame cake. In the first circle, estimate how much the individual who hurt you was to blame for what happened. It will probably be close to 100 per cent. In the next circle think about the other things that might have influenced your reaction, e.g. the fact that you were sad about your cancer, or the ineptitude of friends or medical staff, or problems at work, and see how far you can reduce the blame share of the person you're angry with.

Simon Darnley said: 'People need to ask themselves what life was like before the person hurt them. Often they describe an idealized picture of how things were before – as if everything which is wrong in their lives has happened since that incident.'

Some stress experts also believe you need to understand why the other person behaved in the way which upset you. The point of the exercise is to forgive them, so that although you may occasionally still feel angry, you are liberated from your obsessive resentment.

To do this, you need to separate the person from the event which caused you to be so hurt, and realize that he or she is an inadequate, fallible human being, who can make mistakes, just like anyone else.

Try to understand what might have been going on in that person's mind when the event occurred. Did the hurt occur because the person was deliberately malicious, or perhaps because they were unthinking, or even a little stupid? Is it worth being upset for a long period over someone with these failings? If, on careful reflection and analysis, you conclude the person was deliberately malicious, you need to ask whether you are now unwittingly helping that person to continue to harm you.

FEAR OF RECURRENCE

George, 75, was treated for bladder cancer a couple of years ago. He echoes nearly everyone's feelings when he says: 'The thought that my cancer may return is always there, somewhere at the back of my mind. I try not to worry about it though, because worrying doesn't help.'

It is natural to be fearful that the cancer will return, with fatal results. However, because death is still a taboo subject, many people do not talk about it. As a result, they fail to realize that most of us find it hard to come to terms with the idea of our own death. If your family finds this topic difficult as well, you may need to find a support group that offers you the freedom to talk with others who are in the same situation.

Kathleen Sheridan Russell says: 'People are often tremendously relieved to air these fears, and to discover how many other people share them. However, the nature of people's fears about death are different. Sometimes they will fear that they will die before they achieve what they wanted to do in their lives; sometimes they are worried about the welfare of the people they are leaving behind.

'I always ask people what, specifically, they are worried about, and then we see what we can do to relieve those worries. Sometimes the answer is as simple as sorting out family photographs, or making a will, or returning letters to the sender. Some people simply want to leave everything neat and tidy. But they are afraid that if they do those things, it looks as if they are thinking negatively and giving up.' However, Kathleen says that this type of 'housekeeping' makes no difference to the final outcome and often provides peace of mind.

Fear of a recurrence can also prevent people from planning for the future. It is almost as if they fear that in doing so, they will put a curse on themselves.

Sally, 55, whose cancer was diagnosed five years ago, remembers the early months when she did not dare to keep a box of chocolates from one week to the next. 'There were complications after my operation, and I thought that I probably wouldn't make it, and I might as well eat them all up.

'Although this feeling wore off after a while, it was several years before I had the confidence to plan a holiday. But I have planted some trees in the past couple of years, and now I'm enjoying watching them grow.

'Of course, if I get a bad attack of indigestion, I can't help sometimes wondering if this is "It". Or the thought may pop suddenly into my mind that my disease is bound to come back. But it's like any dreadful thought you have – you have to firmly push it away, and refuse to entertain it.

'If the thoughts won't go away, I think that I've had five good years since my cancer was diagnosed, and I might as well make the best of the time I've got left. And then my indigestion, or whatever, gets better, and I forget all about it.'

Debbie said: 'I came to terms with the uncertainty of my situation quite early on because I realized I had no choice. But breast cancer is continuously on my mind, and not a day goes past when I don't remind myself of what has happened. I still find it difficult to plan for holidays, and I look at my garden through very clear glasses. I think I'm at an inbetween phase, and I hope I'm about to move into another stage of recovery.'

John, speaking less than a year after his bowel cancer was diagnosed, said: 'I have decided my cancer is an episode that is now over, and I'm going to carry on as normal. I do sometimes think about recurrence, of course I do. But I will meet it when and if it happens. I don't believe in building walls to climb over.'

CHAPTER 9

COMPLEMENTARY THERAPIES

Visualization is a very powerful technique, provided it is used in the right way. I think the right way means using it to tell yourself you feel stronger and better and that you have more energy.

DR MAURICE SLEVIN

CONVENTIONAL VERSUS COMPLEMENTARY

Imagine the scene: in a small corner of the country, a spiritual healer is curing one person with cancer, and then another, and then another. After three months, everyone who has cancer for miles around has been cured, and the story has made news worldwide.

Imagine another scene: in an undistinguished local hospital a young doctor is trying out a new combination of drugs and immune-boosting therapies, and every cancer patient who tries it is cured. Patients from miles around get to hear of the doctor's success and demand to be sent to the hospital. Queues of desperate people form in hospital corridors, the switchboard is jammed, and the story makes news worldwide.

Occasionally we read stories in newspapers that appear to echo those two scenarios, but then, somehow, they peter out. After a while, the healer's patients start to die off at the same rate as those who were not treated. The conventional wonder treatment turns out to work only for one very specialized form of cancer.

Whatever claims are made, whatever you read, neither alternative medicine nor conventional medicine offers any guarantees of curing your cancer. Perhaps, this inability to guarantee success explains why conventional and alternative practitioners are so critical of each other (sometimes to the point of slander).

The conventionally trained doctor argues that his own practice has been carefully evaluated in clinical trials. And while it is true that many clinical treatments offer a survival advantage compared with doing nothing, the advantages of mainstream medicine are sometimes measured in percentages that seem small to the patient. Nevertheless, clinical research is useful, and when the results are translated into medical practice, then some people's lives are saved.

But sometimes the research points doctors in the wrong direction, and it is only after months or years of using a certain treatment that they realize it is not nearly as effective as they hoped. Turning round the juggernaut and persuading doctors to change the way they practise can take a long time. No one practising in the area of cancer can afford to be complacent about what he or she is doing.

A TWENTIETH-CENTURY DISEASE?

You may have seen headlines stating that cancer is on the increase, and this is undoubtedly true. You may have read that this is some twentieth-century evil, caused by our unnatural, stressed and polluted environment. It is then suggested that treatments for cancer lie with natural remedies that provide detoxification, or purification, or boost the immune system, such as coffee enemas, liver herb tonics, laetrile (a derivative of bitter almonds) and iscador (derived from mistletoe).

In fact, the main reason for the increase (apart from avoidable, tobacco-related deaths) is that the population itself is ageing. As we grow older, our immune systems become weaker, and our cellular repair mechanisms become less efficient, increasing our personal risks of contracting cancer. Most mammals living in the wild do not survive long enough to get cancer, but those that do achieve old age are also likely to develop tumours.

Living in a developed country, as we move towards the twenty-first century, is a better time to have cancer than it was in our grandparents' and great-grandparents' time. In the early 1900s, few cancer patients had any hope of long-term survival. Thirty years later, fewer than one in five was alive five years after treatment. In the 1940s, it was one in four, and 20 years later, it was one in three.

Now the American Cancer Society estimates that four out of ten patients who get cancer this year will be alive five years after diagnosis. However, although six out of ten will be dead, many of these will have died from unrelated causes, such as heart disease and stroke (remember, the majority of cancer patients are in the older age groups). When adjustments are made for these factors, it becomes clear that one person in two is now surviving a cancer diagnosis for at least five years.

This five-year figure is frequently quoted as an across-the-board method of evaluating cancer success. For some types of cancer, being clear after five years means you have beaten the disease, but for others, there is still a chance that it will recur later.

COMPARING RESULTS

Complementary therapy can seldom be evaluated in the same way as mainstream medicine. When a new cancer treatment is tested, patients are randomly assigned to receive the new therapy, or another, well-established treatment.

However, cancer patients seek a particular type of complementary therapy because they want to try it. Some of them have exhausted all the cures that mainstream medicine can offer. They would not take kindly to the prospect of being randomly assigned to something entirely different.

All this means that while some complementary therapies are evaluated to similar standards as medical practice, most are not. Your complementary therapist can sometimes quote the results of clinical trials supporting his or her case. However, these trials are unlikely to be as numerous, involve as many patients or survive scientific scrutiny as well as the trials your conventional doctor may be able to pull out of a database. This may not matter too much if they help you as an individual, and are not prohibitively expensive.

Complementary therapies are so called because they do not interfere with mainstream medical treatments. However, anyone with cancer has the right to turn his or her back on orthodox medicine and take an alternative path. This decision may be made because no more curative treatments are on offer, or because the patient is disillusioned with mainstream medicine.

YOUR BODY, YOUR CHOICE

It is your body, and your life, and you may feel that taking control in this way makes you feel happier and stronger. However, there is no evidence that choosing alternative therapies will help you live longer, and some doctors believe that where medical alternatives exist, such a decision will actually shorten your life.

This is a controversial issue where both sides give in to the temptation of publication bias and anecdote. Doctors will tell gruesome stories about patients with 'fungating tumours' beyond all hope of treatment, while the alternative therapists will describe an exceptional individual's miracle cure, as if it applies to everyone. Nevertheless, there is some consensus about the value of complementary therapies that work alongside conventional medicine.

However, if you feel you have had more than enough treatment from the hospital, you may wonder why anyone bothers with complementary therapies. In fact, many people benefit tremendously from them while many others, including most of the people interviewed for this book, never get round to trying them.

COMPLEMENTARY THERAPIES IN HOSPITAL

One reason why complementary therapy is worth considering is that the arch cynics, the doctors themselves, are allowing them to be offered in hospital. This represents a major sea change in a group of professionals who ten or 15 years ago dismissed anything that was not sanctified in a medical textbook or journal as 'mumbo-jumbo'.

In the mid 1970s an American psychiatrist, Dr David Spiegel ,organized a research study to check if weekly support groups would help women with metastatic breast cancer to face their fears of death and dying. The sessions helped the women to communicate better with their doctors, and when the 50 women who attended groups were compared with patients who had not, the attendees had less anxiety, depression, pain and discomfort.

The results were published and that seemed to be that, until ten years later Dr Spiegel decided to follow the women up. He expected the results to show that although the women who attended groups (the treatment group) were better adjusted to their disease, their life expectancy would turn out to be the same as those who did not attend (the control group).

In fact the women who attended the support groups did much better. Of the total of 86 women taking part, 83 had died by the time Dr Spiegel took his second look. All three survivors were in the treatment group, and on average those who had attended the weekly support group had survived for 18 months longer than the controls.

Although the numbers of women involved in this study were fairly small, the results, published in 1989, caused great excitement. Another important aspect of Spiegel's research – the fact that the groups made a significant improvement to the women's quality of life – was almost forgotten.

Other researchers began similar studies, and a revolutionary idea began to creep in. Perhaps cancer patients needed more than a treatment to kill off their cancer cells. And perhaps the cancer-killing treatments would work better if those other needs were addressed. Mainstream doctors began to consider taking a more holistic approach.

GREAT EXPECTATIONS?

Helping people feel better about themselves is not the same as prolonging their lives, yet this point is not always clearly understood by friends and acquaintances. It is also an important issue for you to consider. You may need to decide in your own quest for complementary therapies whether an improved quality of life is enough, or whether you are searching for what so few people can truly offer – a sure-fire cure.

In her book, *Patient No More*, breast cancer patient Sharon Batt describes how she told a stranger at a party that she had been treated for cancer. 'In no time, a small group had gathered to question and advise. One woman told me I should eat garlic; a lot of it, every day. Another asked if I'd heard of a spa for cancer patients in Germany, known for a special diet... Other people probed me gently with questions like, "Are you practising visualizations?"; "Have you made any changes in your life?"; "Do you have a good attitude?" They didn't come right out with it, but the idea was clear: making changes in my life and thinking positively would help me to get better.'

After a year of researching alternative and complementary therapies, Sharon Batt found she had lost interest in understanding why she had got cancer and how she could stop it.

At the same time her obsession with orthodox treatments diminished as well.

She wrote: 'I began to entertain a different view: that curing breast cancer might indeed be a mere wishful fantasy. Although it was frightening, this thought was also liberating. It freed me from a search that had been largely sterile, and enabled me to think about realistic alternatives: ways of living fully with breast cancer and dying of the disease – if it came to that – without the immobilizing fear that leads us to deny the possibility altogether.'

CONFLICTING VIEWS ON YOUR DIET

People who have had cancer probably experience more pressure than any other group to watch what they eat. Doctors now agree that there is wide-scale evidence that a healthy diet can reduce the risks of getting a cancer. The subject of whether it can influence the course of established disease is controversial, and subject to publication bias.

Doctors often cite the example of lung cancer, which is not reversed when the main cause – tobacco – is withdrawn. They do not feel that any number of vitamin supplements, coffee enemas and herbal remedies can reverse faults in the mechanisms that control cell division. Dr Maurice Slevin said: 'I would love to tell patients that they could cure their cancers by changing their diet, but there is not a jot of evidence to support it.'

Dr Slevin is unhappy about the dietary advice offered by Bristol Cancer Help Centre (see below). He explained: 'I'm glad the diet has been modified and now permits some fish and chicken, but even so it advises people to avoid dairy products, which are major sources of nutrition, and salt and sugar which help make foods tasty to a group of people who are often having difficulty in maintaining their weight. I know a lot of doctors are concerned that this eating plan cuts out major components of the diet for no good reason.'

Cancer patients who have lost a lot of weight are advised to eat whatever they can, regardless of whether or not the foods consumed are traditionally viewed as 'healthy'. You may even be encouraged to indulge in such dietary heresies as adding milk powder to full cream milk, slathering butter on your toast and snacking whenever you feel the urge to eat. This is because being significantly underweight is a greater threat to your recovery than the distant prospect of heart disease.

If you are further down the road to recovery, then you will be advised to follow the same healthy diet recommendations as everyone else (see box).

CONVENTIONAL ADVICE FOR A HEALTHY DIET

- Plenty of fruit and vegetables
- Foods high in natural fibre, e.g. wholewheat bread and grains
- More fish and chicken and less red meat
- Less sugar and salt
- Only moderate amounts of tea and coffee
- Moderate amounts of alcohol

THE BRISTOL APPROACH

Some complementary therapists go much further, and argue that people who have had cancer should take special care of their diet. They believe that someone who has been through the shock of cancer diagnosis, and the considerable physical rigours of treatment, needs to pay very special attention to their nourishment.

When Bristol Cancer Help Centre was first opened, many doctors expressed reservations about the strictness of the recommended diet. That diet has now been modified, although it still differs greatly from the way most people choose to eat.

The Bristol diet sheet advises: 'If you decide to make any changes, do so gently, exploring and enjoying the changes rather than feeling under pressure to make them. We are all unique individuals and our nutritional needs are different. The guidelines provided here are generalized and may well need to be modified according to your particular requirements.'

The rationale behind the Bristol diet is that healthy eating will help 'strengthen ourselves physically, emotionally, mentally and spiritually and promote healthy immune and repair functions.'

If you want to try the Bristol diet, which is described below, bear in mind that changes have to be made gradually. This is because if you try to switch overnight from the average Western diet to an eating programme that is high in wholegrain cereals and beans, you will feel windy, bloated and ill.

Try beginning by gradually increasing your fruit and vegetable intake so that you have five servings a day. If you do not already use wholegrain foods, switch to using half white and half brown bread and pastas, and cook with half white and half brown flour. Some people are fairly tolerant of beans (pulses) and lentils, but others will have to introduce them fairly gradually (adding a small can of butter beans to the family casserole for instance).

The soya products that replace dairy foods in the Bristol diet can be very variable in taste and quality. Be prepared to experiment, and ask advice from your local health food shop as to which are the most palatable.

Remember that you are changing your diet to feel better, and not to punish your body for having cancer. If the diet makes you feel better, it is working. Otherwise, it is not. The Bristol guidelines are as follows:

1 Wholefood (i.e. nothing added or taken away), e.g. wholemeal bread, brown flour, brown rice
2 Fresh fruit and vegetables in season, lightly steamed or as salad – try to eat both daily
3 Raw cereals (muesli), nuts, seeds, dried fruits etc. Try to eat some daily
4 Organically grown food, as available and affordable
5 Organic poultry, eggs, game and fish – deep-sea fish is preferable to farmed fish
6 Pulses, i.e. dried beans, peas and lentils. Vegetables and cereals. Bran should be avoided as it is an irritant to the bowel. Pulses should be soaked, then boiled in fresh water for ten minutes, the water should be changed and cooking continued until they are tender. This avoids flatulence and possible toxicity problems
7 Cold pressed oils for cooking and dressings
8 Variety. Avoid excessive dependence on one food
9 Freshly made fruit and vegetable juices using organic fruit and vegetables
10 Up to 2 litres (3+ pints) daily of filtered or spring water, not taken at the same time as meals

The guidelines suggest that, whenever possible, you avoid all chemically farmed fruit, vegetables, meat, fish and eggs. In addition, move towards avoiding the following: red meat; caffeine, i.e. tea, coffee, chocolate, colas; excess alcohol; sugar (use honey and fruit concentrates if necessary); salt; fats and dairy produce (substituting soya alternatives); smoked or pickled foods, preservatives and additives; foods which have been stored for long periods, irradiated, processed, microwaved or repeatedly reheated; margarines and fats/spreads containing hydrogenated fats.

The Bristol Cancer Help Centre also suggests the following supplements for patients in remission:

- Vitamin C – 1gm three times daily
- Beta carotene – 12–15mg daily
- Selenium – 200 micrograms daily
- Vitamin E – 200 international units

IMPORTANT NOTE It has been suggested that vitamin E supplements should not be used by people suffering from hormone-dependent cancers, i.e. of the breast, uterus, ovary, prostate and testis, as it may boost hormone levels. People with high blood pressure or who are taking anti-thrombotic drugs should consult their doctors before taking vitamin E. Vitamin C should not be taken at the same time as the chemotherapy drug, methotrexate.

Some people find their own special diet therapy. Sally, for example, switched to a low-fat diet after developing lymphoedema in both legs. She said: 'I have read that if the lymph system is faulty, it doesn't handle fats very well, and that certainly proved true for me. I get plenty of calories from bread and pasta, and I'm not hungry and not losing weight. I've taught myself to dry fry, not to add fats to bread or dressings to salads, and I feel much better and more energized as a result.'

COMPLEMENTARY THERAPIES: THE MEDICAL VIEW

Psychotherapy, counselling and relaxation are now available from many cancer treatment centres, and are regarded as standard supports for patients. Some centres also offer visualization, massage, aromatherapy, hypnotherapy, self-help groups and art therapy.

There are a number of other complementary therapies that

are not usually offered in hospitals, but which do not cause concern to cancer doctors. These include reflexology, acupuncture, homeopathy, meditation, faith healing and spiritual healing and Bach flower remedies.

Although it is entirely up to you to choose which therapies, if any, you want to pursue, the following therapies are thought by many doctors to be potentially harmful. They include diet therapy, megavitamin therapy, metabolic therapy or immunoaugmentative therapy (using laetrile/iscador/coffee enemas/herb tonics) and herbal remedies. They have become causes for concern because some therapists using these treatments have claimed they can stop cancer growth and produce cures.

RELAXATION AND VISUALIZATION

Relaxation is one of the simplest, cheapest and most accessible therapies available, and it can induce instant calm. Relaxation skills are also needed if you try visualization, autogenic training, self-hypnosis or yoga and so they are described here at some length.

You can learn relaxation from a therapist, use an audiotape or simply read instructions from a book. As you become more proficient, you can add positive suggestions and affirmations to enhance your sense of well-being.

Learning these techniques, and then improving on them, will give you an increased sense of control and achievement. However, you may need to try several different methods before you find one which works for you. If you find that you cannot relax at your allotted time, do not worry. This is not something you can force yourself to do. Simply try again tomorrow.

If you decide to use relaxation you will need to allocate yourself a time (or perhaps two occasions) during the day. Otherwise, perhaps because it is so simple to do, it is easy to keep putting it off.

Until you are familiar with the procedure, you can record your own relaxation tape, based on the instructions below, which come from the BACUP booklet, *Cancer and Complementary Therapies*. Otherwise, you may need to read them two or three times before you start.

If you record, read the instructions slowly, allowing longish pauses between sections. If the timing is wrong when you come to try the exercise, then you can always re-record. You can also buy relaxation audiotapes.

EXERCISE ONE

Find a quiet room where you will be undisturbed for about 10–15 minutes. Undo any tight clothing and remove your shoes, then lie down on the bed or floor. Spend a few moments settling yourself down. Close your eyes, spread your feet 30–45 centimetres (12–18 inches) apart and check that your head, neck and spine are in a straight line.

Now focus your attention on your breathing. Do not try to change your breathing for the moment. Become aware of how fast or slowly you are breathing. Notice whether there are any gaps or pauses between your breathing in and breathing out.

Pause

Now put one hand on your upper chest and one hand on your abdomen just below your rib-cage. Relax your shoulders and hands. As you breathe in, feel your abdomen expand. As you breathe out, allow your abdomen to flatten. There should be little or no movement in your chest. Allow yourself a little time to get into a regular rhythm.

Pause

As you breathe in, imagine you are drawing half a circle with your breath, and as you breathe out, you complete the second half of the circle.

Pause

Allow your breathing to become smooth, easy and regular.

Pause

Now consciously slow down your breathing out and allow your breathing in to follow smoothly and easily.

Pause

Smooth out any gaps or pauses in your breathing.

Pause

If any distractions, thoughts or worries come into your mind, allow them to come, then allow them to go and bring your attention back to your breathing.

Pause

When you are ready to end this exercise, take a few deeper breaths in. Bring some feeling back into your fingers and toes.

Open your eyes slowly and turn on to one side before gently sitting up.

EXERCISE TWO

Find a quiet room where you will be undisturbed for about 10–15 minutes. Undo any tight clothing and remove your shoes, then lie down on the bed or floor. Spend a few moments settling yourself down. Close your eyes, spread your feet 30–45 centimetres (12–18 inches) apart and check that your head, neck and spine are in a straight line.

Starting with your forehead and face, let go of any tension. Relax the muscles of your face and jaw. Check that your teeth are not clenched. Allow your tongue to lie away from the roof of your mouth.

Allow your head and shoulders to fall back easily on the floor or bed. Relax your upper arms, lower arms, hands and fingers. Let go of any tension in your chest and abdomen. Breathe smoothly, regularly, rhythmically and without effort, letting your abdomen expand as you breathe in, and flatten as you breathe out.

Pause

Relax the muscles of your feet, legs and thighs and allow your whole body to be supported by the floor, and focus your attention on your breathing.

Pause

If any thoughts, worries or concerns come into your mind, allow them to come, then allow them to go, bringing your attention back to your breathing.

Pause

When you are ready to finish, bring some feeling back into your fingers and toes – take a few deeper breaths in. Open your eyes gently, turn on to your side and gradually sit up.

Once you realize the benefits of relaxation, you may want to use it at other, odd moments during the day. Here is a quicker exercise, from the American Cancer Society, which you can use when you are sitting.

EXERCISE THREE

Stare at a distant object, or close your eyes and concentrate on your breathing or on a peaceful scene.

Take a slow, deep breath, and, as you breathe in, tense your arm muscles.

As you breathe out, relax your muscles and feel the tension draining.

Now remain relaxed and begin breathing slowly and comfortably, concentrating on your breathing. Do not breathe too deeply.

To maintain a slow, even rhythm as you breathe out, you can say silently, 'In, one, two; out, one, two.' Each time you breathe out, feel yourself relaxing and going limp. If some muscles are not relaxed, e.g. in your shoulders, tense them as you breathe in and relax them as you breathe out.

Continue slow rhythmic breathing for anything from a few seconds up to ten minutes.

When you want the session to end, count silently and slowly from one to three. Open your eyes. Say silently to yourself: 'I feel alert and relaxed.' Begin moving about slowly.

Once you have learned to relax, you can augment the effects by using visualization, i.e. allowing your imagination to create mental pictures and situations at will.

In the past, visualization has been used to imagine cancer cells being blasted away by treatment, or by the body's own immune system. Some people still use this approach, while others prefer more gentle images that enhance their sense of well-being. For example, you can imagine yourself lying on a beach with a warm sun heating your body – or picture yourself fit and well and moving freely through a beautiful imaginary landscape.

Visualization can be useful to help you get through future stressful events. For instance, if you are worried about giving a talk to colleagues, or an encounter with a difficult relative, or a new form of treatment, you can imagine yourself in that situation, handling it well.

Try imagining a ball of healing energy – perhaps a white light, forming somewhere in your body. Once you can picture this in your mind's eye, imagine that as you breathe in, you can blow the ball to the part of your body that you want to be healed. When you breathe out, imagine the air moving the ball away from your body, taking with it any painful or uncomfortable feelings. As you repeat this, you may see the ball getting bigger as it takes away more tension and discomfort.

Relaxation will make you much more aware of your body. You will notice when you have started to tense up and be able to correct this.

IMPORTANT NOTE

If you have any lung problems, do check with your doctor before using any technique that requires deep breathing.

Sharon admits that she went overboard on alternative therapies. She said: 'I was already vegetarian, but I switched to decaffeinated coffee, gave up alcohol, took up yoga, transcendental meditation, cycling, relaxation and visualization. In fact, every day I used to lie on the floor, imagining that my insides were an engine and I was going round with an oily rag. I bought a bicycle and I spent hours reading books on philosophy. I didn't go anywhere without taking Aldous Huxley's book, *The Perennial Philosophy*, with me.

'Although it sounds over the top, the alternative stuff was very powerful because it was a way of channelling my desire to get well again. Five years later I still do yoga, and I still cycle, and I still dip into *The Perennial Philosophy*.

HEALERS

Thousands of people offer their services as healers, both within and outside the Christian church. Healers who work outside the church believe that by laying their hands on or near the patient, they can act as channels for healing energy. This allows the regeneration of the patient's own, faulty, self-healing mechanisms.

Christians believe the healing energy comes from God, a Chinese person talks of Qi and an Indian of prana. Spiritualist healers (as opposed to spirit healers) believe that they are taken over by an entity from the spirit world – often someone who lived in a previous age – while they are in their healing trance. Faith healers, another subgroup, may demand proof that the patient trusts in their healing powers.

Anne Woodham, author of the *HEA Guide to Complementary Medicine and Therapies*, commented: 'As a rule, beware of anyone who makes extortionate demands in return for healing, whether of large sums of money, of belief, or of commitment.' Also, as with all other complementary therapists, you should beware of anyone who promises a cure.

Esme, 75, was in hospital, in great pain after a colostomy operation. She said: 'I dragged myself out of bed and painfully made my way down to the desk where the night nurses were assembled. When I begged for a painkiller they told me they would see to me in a while.

'I got back into bed. The pain was so intense I couldn't open my eyes. I just lay there crying. I was vaguely aware of the woman from the next bed standing next to me. Then she started stroking my arm. I couldn't bring myself to speak to her, but she continued to stroke my arm. I became aware that the pain was moving from my belly to my arm. Each stroke of her hand was like a magnet drawing out the pain. I fell into a deep and undisturbed sleep.'

Some general practitioner fundholders are able to send patients to healers at NHS expense, and hospitals, hospices and pain clinics are making increased use of healers.

At present there is no law that states a practitioner of a complementary therapy must be trained, registered, or attached to a regulatory body. However, in the UK, the Institute for Complementary Medicine administers a register that is based on accredited training, external proof of competence, a code of conduct and insurance for public liability (see Useful Addresses, page 149). This has been approved by the Department of Trade and Industry.

CHAPTER 10

FURTHER TREATMENT

*I didn't get any of the side effects I'd been
warned about – no diarrhoea, no vomiting.
The only thing that got me down were the people in the
waiting room constantly moaning about how long they
were being kept waiting!*

KEVIN, TALKING ABOUT HIS TREATMENT FOR TESTICULAR CANCER

WHAT TO EXPECT

The next two chapters of this book are designed to give you an idea of what to expect if you need treatment, or further treatment, for your cancer.

Otherwise, you may prefer to move on to Chapter 12: Recovery – Moving on, see page 144). For information on the effects of treatment on your sexual and emotional life, refer back to Chapter 5 (see page 50).

CHEMOTHERAPY

Chemotherapy drugs are designed to kill cells as they are in the process of dividing. Although any type of cells can be damaged, cancer cells are more vulnerable because they divide particularly quickly. The troublesome side effects of chemotherapy (cytotoxic) drugs are most likely to occur in the parts of the body where normal cells are also dividing rapidly, i.e. the mouth, digestive system, skin, hair and bone marrow.

A one-off dose of chemotherapy is seldom enough to kill all the circulating cancer cells, but larger doses cannot be given without causing havoc to normal, healthy cells. For this reason anti-cancer drugs often have to be given at intervals over several months. The gaps between the courses of drugs are timed to allow damaged normal cells in the body to recover.

Cytotoxic drugs can be used singly or in combination – which is why you may hear your treatment described as a series of initials, such as CMF (cyclophosphamide, methrotrexate and fluorouracil) in breast cancer. Each drug in a combination works in a slightly different way from the others, damaging or interrupting cell multiplication at a different stage. Combined therapies have so far proved very successful in treating Hodgkin's Disease, leukaemia and cancers of the breast, ovary, lung and testis.

However, chemotherapy drugs do not only vary in their action, but also in the way they affect individuals. Thus some people will report 'sailing through' their treatments with nothing but a little extra fatigue, while others will find the same chemotherapy regime a gruelling experience.

Margaret, who was treated for stomach cancer at 37, and then developed breast cancer at 52, said: 'I had two and a half years of chemotherapy for my stomach cancer, and after that I said, never again. But when I developed breast cancer, I changed my mind. It wasn't a pleasant experience, but doctors were able to offer me some much better treatments for the side effects, and these helped a lot.'

Danny, who had a particularly toxic form of chemotherapy for his teratoma when he was 23, also thought he could never contemplate going through it again. Now at 41, he says: 'If I had a recurrence, I would definitely accept chemotherapy. After all, it saved my life last time.'

Debbie, treated for breast cancer, said: 'I thought the chemo would be terrible, but in fact I was able to have it in the morning, and go to work in the afternoon.'

SIDE EFFECTS OF CHEMOTHERAPY

The list of possible side effects from chemotherapy is long and rather daunting: most of them will never affect you.

Those that do can often be minimized with prompt treatment, and advice from your local cancer unit.

People having chemotherapy realize they are trading a period of discomfort for the hope of a cure, or at least a longer life.

Nevertheless, you need all your physical energy to fight the disease, so do not be too stoical about any unpleasant symptoms caused by your treatment. Your recovery will be delayed if you become debilitated by drug side effects. The best way you can help yourself at this difficult stage is to tell your doctor about any symptoms and be prepared to take whatever is prescribed to relieve them.

Some anti-cancer drugs irritate the bladder, and damage your kidneys and you will need to check with your doctor whether your medication has this effect. The warning signs include pain or burning on urination, increased frequency of urination and often an inability to wait (urgency), reddish or bloody urine, fever and chills.

Don't worry if your urine changes to a bright orange, red or yellow colour, or smells like medicine, or if your semen is similarly affected. Do check these symptoms with your doctor, who will probably be able to reassure you that they are a normal side effect.

Chemotherapy can make your skin dry, slightly discoloured and more sensitive to sunlight. During this time you may need to apply moisturizing creams lavishly and use sunblocks to prevent sunburn. Your nails may grow more slowly, split, or develop white ridges.

Treatments for certain lymphomas and leukaemia may lead to a build up of uric acid in the blood, leading to an increased risk of developing kidney stones or gout. To avoid this, the drug allopurinol is usually given to patients about 24 hours before chemotherapy commences.

Sometimes chemotherapy can affect your mouth, so that food may temporarily taste more salty, bitter or metallic, or you may be left with a sore mouth or mouth ulcers. If you develop a sore mouth or mouth ulcers, you will need to be particularly careful about dental hygiene, and very gentle in the way you treat the skin inside your mouth. You should clean your teeth with a soft-bristled or child's toothbrush every morning and evening, and after each meal. You can increase the softness of the bristles by soaking the brush in hot water before you clean, and rinsing it in the hot water while brushing. If this is just too painful, you could try gauze wrapped round a cotton wool bud. Even if you can't brush your teeth as vigorously as usual, the fluoride in the toothpaste will help protect against cavities. Dental floss is also useful for reaching food particles between the teeth.

If your toothpaste stings, or the taste makes you feel nauseous, try a bicarb mouthwash instead (one teaspoon of bicarbonate of soda dissolved in a mug of warm water). Commercial mouthwashes, which contain a large amount of salt or alcohol, may be too strong. If you have dentures you will need to remove and clean them every morning, evening and after each meal.

Add sauces and gravies to your food to make swallowing easier and try to drink at least 1½ litres (3 pints) of liquid a day. Neat spirits, tobacco, hot spices, garlic, onion, vinegar, lemon juice and salty food are likely to make the problem worse, and are best avoided. Chilled foods, e.g. yoghurt straight from the fridge, and ice cubes and ice cream are helpful. Keep your lips moist by using Vaseline or a lip balm. Tell your doctor about your mouth ulcers, as he or she may be able to prescribe a drug treatment to make eating, talking (and smiling) less painful and avoid mouth infection. It needs to be taken every four hours (so you have to set your alarm for the middle of the night).

Fluid retention can be another annoying side effect that can be caused by hormonal changes resulting from your drugs, or as a direct side effect. Your doctor may advise you to avoid table salt and foods high in sodium, or in more severe cases, prescribe a diuretic.

CHEMOTHERAPY AND BLOOD CELLS

Anti-cancer drugs often have important, but temporary, effects on your bone marrow. Most of our blood cells are manufactured within the bone marrow and then released into the circulation. Damage to the bone marrow can result in problems with the three main types of blood cells: red cells, white cells and platelets.

Red blood cells carry oxygen round the body. If the red cell count drops too low you may notice the symptoms of anaemia – you feel weak, lethargic, dizzy, chilled and short of breath. However, doctors are aware of this risk, and your red cell count should be regularly checked.

If these symptoms appear between checks, then be sure to tell your doctor. You will need to make sure you get plenty of rest until your blood count recovers, and to get up slowly when you are sitting or lying. You may also need a blood transfusion. We are constantly exposed to viruses and bacteria, but only become ill when our natural defences fail to overwhelm the intruding organisms.

White cells play an essential role in destroying invading bugs. If the white-cell count drops below a certain level, our risks of going down with an infection increase. This should be detected from blood tests – and it may be necessary to postpone your next treatment, change your drugs or reduce the dose.

The damaging effects of chemotherapy on white-cell count can be minimized by injections of colony-stimulating factors. These are described in the section on intensive chemotherapy, see page 132.

If you know your white count is low, you will need to be scrupulous about personal hygiene because you will find it hard to withstand even a trivial infection. This means staying away from crowds and avoiding children who have just been immunized or anyone with an infectious disease.

Sometimes, despite your best efforts, you may still get an infection. Warning signs include a high temperature, chills, sweating, a burning feeling when you urinate, a severe cough or sore throat, unusual vaginal discharge or itching, and redness, swelling or tenderness, especially around vulnerable areas such as a wound, sore, pimple, or intravenous catheter site. Some people develop flu-like symptoms – muscle aches, headache, tiredness, nausea, a slight fever, chills and poor appetite – soon after their chemotherapy. These symptoms may be caused by the drugs, or by an infection. If this happens, inform your doctor and do not use drugs (not even aspirin) until you have been given the go-ahead. See also boxed warning (page 128).

Platelets, the smallest of the blood cells, can also be destroyed by chemotherapy. If your platelet count drops too low, you will bruise very easily, and bleed profusely from minor cuts or grazes. In this case, a special type of transfusion, involving platelets only, will be given. Again, you need to take special care with your health, accidental cuts or nicks from scissors, needles, knives or tools (perhaps by avoiding using them at this time), or burns during cooking, ironing or tending a fire or injuries from contact sports. Use a very soft toothbrush, and make sure you blow your nose gently. Over-the-counter drugs, including aspirin and ibuprofen, should be avoided as they can affect your platelet function, along with alcohol.

> ## WARNING
>
> Inform your doctor quickly if you develop a fever (temperature over 38°C/100.4°F) or notice any sign of bleeding or bruising while you are having chemotherapy, or in the rest period after treatment. It could be a sign that your bone marrow is being affected. If you develop an infection you may need hospital admission for intensive antibiotic treatment.

SICKNESS AND NAUSEA

If you are very sick or nauseous, you should inform your doctor and ask if any of the newer anti-sickness drugs would be helpful next time. Some hospitals provide these as a matter of course while others tend to economize by only giving those to patients who suffer most (or shout loudest).

Ondansetron, granisetron and tropisetron are fairly new (and therefore expensive) drugs that are particularly effective with the cancer drugs which cause the most severe sickness. They need to be given in the very early stages of sickness, because they do not work so well once vomiting is well established, e.g. after it has been going on for 24 hours or more.

Less severe nausea and sickness are often treated with prochlorperazine, domperidone, dexamethasone and/or lorazepam. These drugs are often given before and after chemotherapy.

Whether you are having chemotherapy for the first time or not, it may be to your advantage to discuss what remedies are available for nausea and sickness. You may be reassured that your particular drug regimen causes few or mild symptoms. However, if you discover you are on one of the more toxic therapies, it is worth emphasizing your dislike of being sick and nauseous.

Some people who have had a bad time with chemotherapy feel sick when they cross the threshold of the hospital – or even if they watch a hospital soap. This kind of conditioned response can be hard to deal with, and ideally you should avoid it happening to you.

Hypnosis, self-hypnosis and relaxation therapies can often help, so ask the doctor if these are available. Even if they are not, you are making a point that may be helpful to you next time, or to other patients in future. You can choose from a number of audio tapes which describe these techniques. For more information refer to Chapter 9 (see page 108).

John, diagnosed with bowel cancer at 49, says: 'The first couple of times I had chemotherapy, it was tolerable. As time went on it got harder and harder to drag myself to the hospital. I was having one week on, and three weeks off, and it was difficult to get yourself fit again, while knowing what was coming up in a couple of weeks' time. In the end, I had a lot of sickness and diarrhoea, and had to force myself to go to the hospital. It reached the point where even the smell of a hospital made me feel sick.'

If your nausea persists, despite the drugs prescribed by your doctor, you could try shifting to a grazing pattern of eating. This involves frequent small meals or snacks during the day (including bedtime). Rest in a chair after eating, but try to avoid lying flat for at least two hours after a meal.

Many people develop a dislike for the taste of red meat, but are still able to tolerate fish and chicken meals. Lemon drops or mint sweets that leave a pleasant aroma in the mouth are helpful, and you may sometimes find it is easier to eat cold foods that smell less strong than a meal that comes steaming from the cooker or microwave.

It can be infuriating to have the world urging you to eat well and keep your strength up, when this is physically impossible. If you can't keep down much food, promise yourself you will make a special effort to eat well when the nausea has worn off (even if you still don't feel like it).

If you are being sick, it is important to avoid dehydration, so choose clear liquids (water and drinks that you can see through such as ginger ale, some apple juices, tea, etc.). You may find it easier to take liquids in the form of ice chips. If you have a bad bout of vomiting, do not try to eat for at least four to eight hours, and then start with clear liquids.

Contact your doctor if you are too sick to take your medication (when suppositories or injections will be given instead); if you vomit more than three times an hour for three or more hours; if any blood or material that looks like coffee grounds appear in the vomit; if you suspect that you have inhaled vomited material; if you are unable to take in more than four cups of liquid in a day, or are unable to eat solid foods for more than two days.

Weakness and dizziness often occur after vomiting, but if they persist you should inform your doctor. If there is a danger that vomiting will occur while you are asleep, make sure you lie on your side or front to avoid accidentally inhaling vomit.

If you want to try an alternative, then some people find that Sea-Bands, generally used for seasickness, can be very helpful with chemotherapy-induced nausea. These can be used along with any other medications you may take to control side effects, or as an alternative, and they have no side effects. The device works on the ancient Chinese principle of acupressure and consists of an elastic wristband with a plastic stud that applies pressure on a special point on the wrist.

Elsie, diagnosed with bowel cancer at 58, said: 'I had to have chemotherapy injections every week for six months, and they made me sick to the stomach. Then the nurses offered me a change of anti-emetic drug, along with these acupressure bands. I was sceptical at first, but they certainly worked for me.

'I get my chemo on a Tuesday, and take the anti-sickness drugs then. I keep the bands on until Wednesday night, and after that, if I feel queasy, I don't take any more anti-sickness drugs, I just apply a little extra pressure on each wrist. It certainly works for me and it's a pity more people don't know about it.'

Chemotherapy can also damage the cells in the lining of the stomach and intestine, causing digestive disorders such as diarrhoea, and less commonly, constipation. More details on how to cope with these conditions are given in Chapter 11 (see page 134).

HAIR LOSS AND THINNING

Chemotherapy can damage the hair follicles, causing hair loss, although not all drugs have this effect. But even if you have been warned that you are likely to lose your hair, finding handfuls on the pillow, or in your hairbrush can be a shock. Hair loss starts to occur within two weeks of the start of treatment, and gets worse one to two months later.

Unfortunately, there is no effective treatment for hair loss, but you can expect your hair to grow back. Sometimes, however, the new hair is a different colour or is more or less straight. In some hospitals, patients are offered the chance to wear an ice cold cap on their heads, to constrict the blood vessels serving the scalp and limit the amount of the drug taken up by the hair follicles.

If you are expecting to lose your hair, make an early appointment for a wig fitting (provided on the NHS and frequently covered by insurance in the US) so that you can achieve a close match to the colour and texture of your real hair. You may also find it easier than trying on wigs after you have lost your own hair. Some people wear their wigs during their waking hours, while others find they feel like actors in a play, and prefer turbans, scarves or caps.

Having your hair cut short may help ease the transition to baldness. If your drugs cause thinning rather than total loss, it is also worth cutting your hair because the weight of long hair pulling on the scalp can increase the rate of loss. Shorter styles make the hair look thicker.

Use mild shampoos and soft hair brushes, use hair dryers on the cool setting (or avoid using them altogether), and also avoid hair dyes, perms and rollers.

Samantha, diagnosed with breast cancer at 24, says: 'I had been warned my hair would fall out, and I got it cut very short just beforehand so it wouldn't look too bad when it happened. But nothing I could do prepared me for what I would look like. I felt worse than when I was told I had cancer.

'I didn't really like wearing a wig because I thought everyone could tell it wasn't real. So I wore a basketball cap during the day and kept the wig for evenings when I was going out. I got quite upset when people stared at me in my baseball cap. It looked as if my head was shaved underneath. But then I realized I would probably have stared as well. My hair regrew when I stopped the treatment.'

RISKS OF TREATMENT

Cancer specialists must always weigh the benefits of a drug that might save a patient's life against the drawbacks. Some of the more powerful cancer drugs can cause damage to the kidneys, hearing loss, tinnitus and damage to the peripheral nervous system. These include the class of drugs known as the vinca alkaloids, e.g. vincristine, for leukaemia, lymphoma and breast and lung cancer; cisplatin, for ovarian cancer and testicular cancer; and paclitaxel, for metastatic ovarian cancer and breast cancer.

The use of these toxic drugs is carefully monitored so doses can be withdrawn, or treatment ceased. Cancer specialists vary as individuals, and from country to country, as to how 'aggressive' they are prepared to be in the use of such drugs in the battle against a life-threatening disease. In general, American oncologists are regarded as being more aggressive than their European counterparts. However regardless of who is treating you, you should expect to be fully informed of the risks you take when this type of treatment is prescribed.

Despite these precautions some people are left with peripheral neuropathy – damage to the nerves that connect the central nervous system to the sense organs, muscles, glands and internal organs. The symptoms include tingling, burning, weakness or numbness in the hands or feet, loss of balance, clumsiness, difficulty in picking up objects and buttoning clothing, walking problems, jaw pain, hearing loss, stomach pain and constipation. These symptoms are sometimes transient, but unfortunately they can be permanent, and you may need to adjust to living with them. They should, of course, be reported to your doctor.

INTENSIVE CHEMOTHERAPY

Chemotherapy drugs can destroy the blood-forming cells in the bone marrow, and for that reason doses have to be limited. Otherwise, the patient is killed along with the cancer. Several developments have now made it possible to give much higher doses, sometimes accompanied by irradiation of the whole body, even though this will cause irreparable damage to the bone marrow.

Healthy bone marrow can now be transplanted after treatment with high-dose drug or radiotherapy treatment. Transplants may be autologous (involving the patient's own bone marrow removed before chemotherapy) or from a matched donor.

Chemotherapy damages the white blood cells, leaving the patient vulnerable to infection. This damage can be limited with an injection of a new type of drug, known as colony-stimulating factors (CSF). These stimulate the production of two different types of white blood cell within the bone marrow. Treatment with CSF usually lasts for 7–10 days, and is given after each course of chemotherapy. Some people find that their chemotherapy has to be delayed because of its harmful effects on their blood. The use of CSF treatment makes these delays less likely, as well as allowing higher doses to be given.

Some doctors now believe that peripheral blood stem cells

transplantation may be better than bone marrow transplantation. This procedure involves stimulating the bone marrow to release stem cells (immature blood cells) into the circulation. The stem cells are collected before treatment, and then replaced afterwards.

THE NEXT GENERATION OF DRUGS

There are hundreds of new cancer drugs currently under development. Some of them will eventually represent breakthroughs for people suffering from certain forms of cancer, others will prove to be a disappointment. Their effectiveness can only be established by testing them on patients.

New drugs are very expensive, and if they work, they can make huge profits for the pharmaceutical companies that manufacture them. Most health systems are short of money, and the pharmaceutical manufacturers have to be very persuasive to convince the budget holders of the value of paying for expensive new drugs. They do not exactly lie about what their drugs will do, but sometimes the temptation to exaggerate the results can become irresistible. Sometimes, too, journalists in search of a good story make a small advance in one rather rarefied form of cancer seem as if a cure has been found for everything. Five years later that drug may have become standard treatment, or it may have vanished without trace.

Drugs which are being tested on human patients for the first time can prove to be unexpectedly toxic as well – and some may cause much more harm than good. See the section on clinical trials in Chapter 7 (page 90).

CHAPTER 11

MORE TREATMENTS – MINIMIZING SIDE EFFECTS

I approached radiotherapy thinking that it was blasting away my cancer, and although my mouth was badly burned I felt energized – full of beans.

RENÉE, DIAGNOSED WITH FACIAL CANCER

STEROIDS AND HORMONES

Hormones are chemical messengers that control cell growth and the function of certain organs, e.g. the ovaries in women, the testes in men. Some tumours, particularly those that affect the breast, prostate, thyroid and womb, are particularly responsive to hormonal influences.

If the body's hormonal climate is changed, the tumours may stop growing or shrink. Hormone therapy is a much gentler treatment than cytotoxic treatments, but it is not always easy to predict whether or not it will work for a particular patient.

Hormone therapy (also known as hormonal manipulation) sometimes involves destroying or removing the gland that produces a particular hormone, e.g. by removing the ovaries to curtail the production of the female hormone, oestrogen. Another approach is to use a drug treatment to block the action of a hormone, e.g. goserelin, which works on the pituitary gland to reduce production of the male hormone, testosterone. Very large doses of hormones can also sometimes stop the growth of tumour cells.

Treatments that involve manipulation of the sex hormones

can cause problems such as temporary impotence, loss of sexual desire, breast swelling in men, and menopausal symptoms and increased risk of thrombosis in women.

The most widely prescribed hormone treatment currently available is tamoxifen, which partially blocks the effects of oestrogen. This is used both as a treatment for breast cancer and in the prevention of recurrence of the disease.

If you are prescribed hormones for the first time, it is important to ask what side effects you should expect and whether there are any warning signs you should watch for, e.g. calf pain in a woman treated with high-dose oestrogens could signify thrombosis.

Another type of hormone, corticosteroids, are used to relieve symptoms such as nausea and poor appetite and reduce swelling caused by cancer deposits in the brain. If you are taking corticosteroids you may notice distressing but temporary problems such as insomnia, muscle weakness and increases in facial hair, urination, thirst and appetite. One of the most annoying side effects is the increase in fat on the cheeks, leading to the typical 'moon-faced' look, and also on the abdomen and back of the neck. Sometimes you and your doctor may have to balance the advantages of taking steroids to relieve your symptoms against the side effects.

Samantha, 24, experienced problems with the steroids given to help counteract the sickness caused by chemotherapy for breast cancer. 'They made me really energetic and rather aggressive and hard to live with. And I also put on a lot of weight because my appetite was so huge and that got me down. In the end, I managed my last lot of chemo without them – although it made me very sick.'

In men oestrogen therapy can cause swelling of the breasts, a loss in sexual interest, and a more youthful appearance (caused by changes in the texture of the facial skin). In women oestrogens can cause fluid retention and vaginal discharge or bleeding. When the male hormone androgen is given to women it can cause fluid retention, increased sexual interest, an increase in facial hair and the loss of scalp hair, and increases in muscle size. Tamoxifen can cause menopausal symptoms such as hot flushes (flashes) and vaginal dryness, while progesterone can cause fluid retention and vaginal discharge. Remember these side effects are temporary and will be reversed once your therapy is completed.

If your steroids or hormones are causing you distress, carry on taking the tablets, but get medical advice as soon as possible. Abruptly stopping certain of these therapies can make you feel even worse, and the sudden cessation of corticosteroid treatment can be dangerous.

You should inform your doctor of any unpleasant symptoms but particularly if you have the following: vomiting, insomnia, shortness of breath, dehydration, fever, black stools, excessive urination or pain, or mood swings which are disturbing you or others.

RADIOTHERAPY

Cancers cannot always be cut away, and so radiotherapy (radiation treatment) is used to destroy the tumour cells on site. The x-rays used in radiotherapy have sufficient energy to disrupt human tissues. Just as tumour cells are more sensitive than normal cells to chemotherapy, they are also more sensitive to radiotherapy. And as with chemotherapy, the difference between a dose that harms the patients and a dose that helps is a fine one. Although radiotherapy can produce a number of side effects, most of them are temporary and can be treated.

Radiotherapy is usually given in a number of small treatments or fractions for up to five days a week, for two to six weeks. It can be given externally, or internally, before, during or after surgery, with or instead of chemotherapy and also as a high-dose treatment when combined with a bone marrow transplant.

Research is now under way to see if giving radiotherapy treatment twice or three times a day, for a shorter period of time, is more effective than a once-a-day approach.

Finding yourself alone in a basement room with a huge radiotherapy machine can be very daunting, but treatment usually lasts only a few minutes at a time.

Radiotherapy may be used to attempt to cure your cancer, or to shrink down your tumour so that it can be destroyed by surgery or chemotherapy, or to relieve your symptoms and improve your quality and length of life.

POSSIBLE SIDE EFFECTS

You should ask your radiotherapist what he or she hopes to achieve with your treatment, and any likely side effects.

Tiredness, caused by the effects of radiation on normal cells, is a common symptom that can creep up on you as your radiotherapy progresses, so if you had planned to work, you may need to take some time off to recover. If you are at home, you may need help with the chores. Fatigue can continue for four to six weeks after treatment ends.

You also need to take special care of the skin in the treatment field. The sweat glands in the irradiated area stop working during treatment, so perspiration is not a problem. Some radiotherapists ask you not to put anything on your skin at this time, because many products leave a coating that can interfere with radiation therapy or healing, while others allow a dusting of mild baby powder three or four times a day.

SKIN CARE

In the treated area:
- Avoid extremes of temperature, e.g. hot water bottles, ice packs
- If necessary, splash with lukewarm water
- Do not rub or scrub treated skin
- Do not use any creams, lotions, perfumes, talc, deodorant or any other substance unless recommended by your doctor
- Avoid shaving
- Wear loose, soft clothing over the treated area
- Protect your skin from the sun by covering, or ask your doctor to recommend a sunblock
- Skin needs to be protected from sunlight for at least a year after treatment

A few weeks after your therapy ends, you may find your skin becomes very dry and itchy. Sometimes a 'moist reaction' can occur, especially in skin folds, and your doctor will need to prescribe a special cream to avoid the risk of infection.

Hair loss occurs only in the treated area, and can be lost from the scalp, face or body. If the radiation is palliative (designed to relieve symptoms rather than cure), then the hair is likely to grow back. If it is curative, then the hair may not return because of the large size of the dose given, or the hair that does regrow may be very fine. You need to ask your doctor about the likely consequences to your own hair. More information about hair loss is given in the section on chemotherapy (see page 130).

Radiotherapy can affect your blood, leading to low white-cell or platelet counts. Because this can affect your ability to fight infection, and your blood-clotting mechanisms, it may be necessary to delay your treatment for a few days.

LOCALIZED SIDE EFFECTS OF RADIOTHERAPY

According to where the radiotherapy was given, other side effects may occur. If you have radiotherapy to your head and/or neck you may find your mouth becomes dry, making swallowing difficult. This is because of damage to the salivary glands, and you may find it helpful to carry a large cup or bottle of water with you during the day, and to keep water by your bedside. Fizzy drinks may also help, along with sugar-free candy or gum (avoid sugar because your teeth are particularly vulnerable to cavities at this time).

This problem does not always clear up after treatment, and you may need to be prescribed an artificial saliva spray. While your mouth is dry you are at increased risk of mouth infections such as thrush, which may require treatment. You also need to take extra care when cleaning your teeth, and with general dental hygiene, as described in the chemotherapy section (see page 125).

Food can taste metallic, or lose its taste completely, although this symptom usually clears up after a few weeks. Your dentures may no longer fit so well, because radiation has caused your gums to swell.

You may also notice earache caused by hardening of the ear wax, and swelling or dropping of the skin under your chin.

Loss of appetite, especially if you have a painful mouth, is common and understandable, but needs to be treated, so tell your doctor immediately. More information on how to cope with this is given on page 143.

Renée suffered severe burns to the inside of her mouth following radiotherapy for her facial cancer. Her radiotherapy was given while she was wearing a special fixed mould, which covered her face. She said: 'The mould was a bit unpleasant, but it was only for a couple of minutes and I focused on the fact that the treatment was making me better.

'I was told I might be sick, but I said very firmly that I was not going to be – and I wasn't. It was the same when I was warned that my loss of taste and smell would be permanent. I didn't believe it, and I was right. I think if you get worked up about symptoms, then they will happen. It's true that eating was painful from halfway through the treatment until about three weeks afterwards. I lost 2½ stones [35lb/16kg], but I was quite pleased about that because I'd needed to lose some weight.'

Radiation to the chest and thorax causes problems in swallowing, which you may mistake for a cancer symptom. In fact they are a common reaction to treatment. You will probably be advised to switch to a soft-food diet, supplemented by drinks designed to build you up, e.g. Complan. You may need painkillers, liquid medicines or gargles containing aspirin before meals to make eating easier. The soreness usually gets better in about five to eight days.

If you develop a cough or shortness of breath, you should tell your doctor, as it may be necessary to adjust your therapy. Patients treated for breast cancer can develop shoulder stiffness, and you may need to be shown exercises to keep your arm moving freely. You should also tell your doctor about any build-up of fluid in the treated area.

Nausea and vomiting can occur after radiotherapy to the chest, thorax, abdomen and pelvis and is common when the treatment area is near the stomach. It may help to avoid eating for a few hours before treatment, and to wait one or two hours afterwards before tackling food. If the problem persists, you may need to be prescribed an anti-sickness drug. For suggestions on how to cope with nausea and vomiting see pages 128–30.

Diarrhoea, stomach cramps and wind are common side effects for people who have radiotherapy to the abdomen and pelvis. Symptoms may disappear quickly or linger for weeks. Your doctor can prescribe anti-diarrhoeal remedies, and should be informed if they don't work. For more information on controlling diarrhoea see page 141.

Painkillers

The use of painkillers arouses surprisingly strong emotions: some people have no qualms about reaching for the aspirin bottle at the first hint of a headache, while others make a virtue of a life free of analgesics. Medically, there is no contest between these arguments. The best way of controlling pain is to treat it before it has a chance to take hold. Although you are taking your medication fairly often this way, you can probably use a lower dose than if you wait until the pain gets bad.

If your doctor has told you that paracetamol, ibuprofen (or acetaminophen) should control your pain, you may wonder why you are being fobbed off with a treatment you can buy without prescription. In fact these drugs are stronger than most people realize, and for mild to moderate pain can be as effective as some prescription pain relievers.

Sometimes, you may find that at first the painkiller is strong enough but the pain returns before you are due to take your next lot of medication. As soon as this happens, contact your doctor to check if you can take your medication more frequently or if you need to move on to something else.

If you need something stronger and are prescribed codeine, or one of its derivatives, it is worth asking for a laxative at the same time as these are very constipating. Otherwise, prescription-only versions of a non-steroidal anti-inflammatory drug may be suggested. These are particularly useful when cancer has spread into the bones.

If your prescribed drugs have failed to control your pain, your doctor is likely to prescribe a long-lasting version of the drug morphine, which can be given twice a day. There is tremendous variation between individuals in the amount of morphine they need, and some people want a larger dose to get through a busy day than they require at night. Morphine can cause nausea and vomiting for the first few days. The symptoms are rather like travel sickness, and it may help to stay in bed for an hour or so after you take your medication. Your doctor may also prescribe an anti-sickness drug.

It is likely that you will also be given laxatives to take regularly as nearly everyone on morphine has constipation. You can help yourself by increasing the fibre in your diet and adding bran to meals. Drinking eight to ten glasses of fluid a day is also helpful.

If your pain is not controlled, despite your doctor's best efforts, ask if you can be referred to a pain specialist. As Dr Maurice Slevin comments: 'None of us can be experts in every aspect of cancer, and sometimes the time comes when we have to hand a patient over to the expertise of a colleague.'

If drugs fail, it may be possible for a surgeon to cut the nerves that are relaying pain impulses to the brain (the same effect can sometimes be achieved with an injection).

However, the solution to pain is not solely medical. It is well known that anxiety, depression and fear can intensify our sensations of pain. The use of relaxation techniques, imagery or skin stimulation – along with your medication – can make an enormous difference to your perception of pain. More information about this is given in Chapter 8 (see page 93).

DIARRHOEA

This complaint can be a nuisance for up to three weeks after treatment with chemotherapy or radiotherapy. It can also be caused by an infection, other drug treatments (apart from chemotherapy), surgery, anxiety, certain food supplements designed to build you up, and as a result of tumour growth.

A grazing style of eating, rather than consuming three meals a day, is helpful. Some people find that adding nutmeg to foods helps slow the intestinal movements. The list of foods that are best avoided is discouragingly long, but remember that for most people, diarrhoea is a temporary nuisance.

Stay away from the kind of high-fibre foods we're normally encouraged to eat, and anything which will irritate the stomach and intestines. This includes dairy products, whole-grain breads and cereals, anything containing bran, nuts, raw fruits, raw vegetables, fried foods, fatty foods (including pastries and confectionary), spicy foods (curries, chilli con carne, etc.), caffeine and alcohol, or food which is very hot or very cold. Good choices at this time include cottage cheese, eggs, mashed or baked potato (without the skin), puréed vegetables, chicken or turkey without the skin, fish, boiled white rice, pasta, canned or cooked fruit without skins, yoghurt, smooth peanut butter and white bread.

Diarrhoea can cause you to run low of potassium, an important mineral. Bananas, oranges, potatoes and peach and apricot nectar are good sources of potassium. You will need extra fluids to avoid dehydration, so it is worth keeping a bottle of water at your side and aiming to drink about 3.5 litres (6 pints a day). However, you need to sip your drinks slowly to avoid overloading the stomach and further irritating the intestine.

If your diarrhoea lasts for more than two days, start a diet of clear liquids, and gradually add foods from the list above. If you are unable to take any solids at all after two days, inform your doctor. You should also inform your doctor if your diarrhoea is severe (i.e. you have more than six to eight loose bowel movements per day for more than two days in a row).

After each bowel movement you may find it helpful to use wet wipes, or mild soap and water to clean your anus, and pat yourself dry. Any soreness can be relieved with a water-repellent cream of the type used for nappy rash. Your doctor may also be able to prescribe a local anaesthetic ointment.

Inform your doctor if you notice blood round your anus (although this is often a result of straining and soreness), or blood in your stools; if you have difficulty with urination; if you cannot take liquids for more than two days; if your abdomen suddenly swells up; if you have a fever; if you lose more than 2kg (5lbs) in weight; or if you notice any new pains (apart from abdominal cramps that precede the diarrhoea).

CONSTIPATION

This can be caused by lack of exercise, not enough food and fluid, some chemotherapy drugs, and pain-relief medication. You are constipated if your bowel movements become much less frequent than is usual for you (for some people a once or twice weekly bowel movement is normal while others may go twice a day); or when your movements involve the passage of hard faeces, and pain and discomfort. Other symptoms include stomach aches or cramps, an excess of wind or belching, an inflated belly, vomiting and nausea.

Constipation is often a temporary annoyance that you can cure yourself by increasing the amount you drink (warm and hot drinks in the morning are particularly helpful) and by increasing the fibre in your diet. Choose from extra bran, wholegrain breads and cereals, vegetables (raw and cooked), fruit (fresh and dried), nuts and popcorn. Don't try to include them all.

Avoid chocolate, cheese and eggs, which can make the problem worse. If you feel up to it, regular exercise will also help solve this problem. Do not use over-the-counter laxatives or self-administered enemas except on medical advice.

Call your doctor if you have not had a bowel movement in

more than three days (unless this is normal for you), if you notice blood around your anus or on your faeces, or if you have persistent cramps and vomiting. You should also inform the doctor if your laxatives have not worked after two days, or if a period of constipation has been followed by oozing of fecal material from your anus. Do not waste the energy you need to fight your cancer on suffering these problems in silence. Treatments are available.

EATING DIFFICULTIES

If your treatment has left your mouth dry and sore, or makes swallowing difficult, some of the following tips may help. If they are easier to eat, indulge yourself in foods that you might normally regard as too calorific or 'unhealthy'. At this stage, any food that helps keep up your calorie intake and rebuilds your strength is a health food.

If you hate soft mushy food, and feel you are being returned to babyhood, remember these problems are nearly always temporary. Cancer treatments don't last for ever, even if they feel as if they do.

The National Cancer Institute of the US also suggests the following:

- Change the consistencies of food by adding more gravies and sauces to make them softer
- Avoid foods that are highly spiced, or have a rough texture such as crisps and crackers
- Eat small, frequent meals
- Cut your food into small, bite-sized pieces
- Ask your doctor if you can take a medicine to ease the pain in your throat before meals
- Tell your doctor if eating solid foods is too difficult – he or she will prescribe liquid supplements instead

CHAPTER 12

RECOVERY – MOVING ON

Samantha, 30 months after her breast cancer diagnosis:
'I do still think about it a lot, and talk about it. I realize it was bad luck that it happened to me – other times I think it happened and it is in the past.'

Danny, diagnosed with testicular teratoma at 23, which recurred 14 years later:
'I know how short life is, and that is double-edged. I worry about worrying sometimes, and then decide I should go with the flow. At other times, I want to cram everything in. I feel I've been very lucky to have survived. Life is too short for relaxation.'

Sylvia, four years after cervical cancer:
'I was ill for quite a while before I was diagnosed, and I'm feeling better than I have for years. Most of the time I can put cancer at the back of my mind. I used to work in a cotton mill, lifting heavy bales, but after I had cancer I thought I've worked all this time, and I've brought up five kids on my own. I'm not going to work any more. And I don't.'

Margaret, diagnosed with stomach cancer at 37 and 15 years later with breast cancer:
'I go for days when I forget all about cancer. I do think it will get me in the end, and having decided that helps to take the fear away. But it's not getting me yet. I've got too much to get done. Cancer hasn't diminished my life – it's taught me to live each day to the full. I'm much more tolerant of people as a result of what I've experienced, and I think I get more out of life from having had these experiences.'

Kevin, a year after testicular cancer:
'Once this has happened to you, then you are never sure what is going to be round the next corner. It was something totally out of the blue, and I feel I've been lucky. It could have caused me a lot of grief, and I know I've got a lot more to look forward to.'

Renée, diagnosed with facial cancer three years ago:
'Losing my nose was something I couldn't change – couldn't do anything about. I decided I was not bloody well going to go under. I think my present nose – the prosthesis – looks better than the original, and my friends are relieved that I make jokes about it. People think it's all so terrible, but it isn't terrible. I can't play tennis any more because of stiffness in my shoulder from the neck operation, but that's not such a loss at my age. I enjoy my life as I did before.'

Sharon, five years after cervical cancer:
'I hardly ever think about having a recurrence now. Sometimes all this stuff about cures turns me off, because you have to die some time. Living while waiting to die would be awful. There's another thing… you have to be careful how you say this, and who you say it to. But the truth is that I would not like to have missed this experience, awful though it was at the time. Even if I die of it in the end, I don't think I will regret having had it. Cancer has given me time to think through my life, to take stock and to sort myself out – and decide what is really important.'

John, a year after diagnosis with bowel cancer:
'I am still testing to see what I can do and what I cannot. I'm back at work full-time, driving the length of the country, but nevertheless, I'm very aware of what I'm doing. If you push yourself too hard your body soon tells you. I've decided to get more out of my leisure time, like going paragliding, for instance. I'm hoping to achieve a better balance between work and pleasure and family life.'

Jean, two years after her breast cancer diagnosis:
'Having a breast reconstruction operation restored my self-esteem and my self-confidence, and I feel it enabled me to start living again. I feel cancer has given me a better perspective on life – and you certainly think twice about saying "yes" all the time.'

Sally, five years after treatment for cervical cancer:
'It has cleared my eyes for all the good things in life, and taught me to live one day at a time. It's also made me less tolerant, because you don't feel you can let things pass. If someone is rude and dismissive to me, for instance in a shop, I will tell them what I think. In the past, I would have let it go. I look at each day with clean eyes, and with each family get-together, I am glad to be there.'

USEFUL ADDRESSES

Please enclose a stamped self-addressed envelope when writing to the organizations below.

UNITED KINGDOM

BACUP

3 Bath Place, Rivington Street, London EC2A 3JR
Tel: 0171 613 2121 if you are ringing from London; 0800 181199 for a free call from outside the 0171 and 0181 telephone districts.

The initials stand for the British Association of Cancer-United Patients. BACUP has a free cancer information service staffed by trained cancer nurses. They provide information, emotional support and practical advice by telephone or letter and can tell you about treatment, research, support groups, therapists, counsellors, financial assistance, insurance, home nursing services and much more. Free booklets are also sent out.

BACUP also runs a free Cancer Counselling Service. Tel: 0171 696 9000 except Scotland; 0141 248 9277 for Scotland.

BRISTOL CANCER HELP CENTRE

Grove House, Cornwallis Grove, Clifton, Bristol, Avon BS8 4PG
Tel: 0117 9743216

Offers a holistic approach to cancer, catering for the mind, body and spirit. Residential or day programmes are available.

BRITISH ASSOCIATION FOR COUNSELLING (BAC)

1 Regent Place, Rugby, Warwickshire CV21 2PJ
Tel: 01788 578328

Can provide a list of trained counsellors throughout the UK, and a fact sheet.

BRITISH INSURANCE AND INVESTMENT BROKERS ASSOCIATION (BIIBA)

BIIBA House, 14 Bevis Marks, London EC3A 7NT
Tel: 0171 623 9043
Offers help finding a broker or local independent financial advisor, and will arrange Travel Special Needs Insurance.

CANCERLINK

17 Britannia Street, London WC1X 9JN
Tel: 0171 833 2451 for England, Wales and Northern Ireland; 0131 228 5557 for Scotland
Offers support and information on all aspects of cancer in response to telephone and letter enquiries, and acts as a resource for hundreds of cancer support and self-help groups throughout the UK.

CANCER RELIEF MACMILLAN FUND

15/19 Britten Street, London SW3 3TZ
Tel: 0171 352 7811
Provides home care nurses and financial grants for people with cancer and their families.

CANCER RESEARCH CAMPAIGN

2 Carlton House Terrace, London SW1Y 5AR
Tel: 0171 930 8972
Funds research into the prevention and cure of cancer, and also has an education programme.

DISABILITY ALLIANCE

1st floor, Universal House, 88–94 Wentworth Street, London E1 7SA
Tel: 0171 247 8763
Provides advice for people with disabilities on welfare benefits and also publishes the *Disability Rights Handbook*.

DSS BENEFITS AGENCY

Tel: 0800 666555 for England, Scotland and Wales; 0800 616757 for Northern Ireland
Provides a confidential freeline phone service giving information on benefits and how to claim them.

IMPERIAL CANCER RESEARCH FUND

PO Box 123, Lincoln's Inn Fields, London WC2A 3PX
Tel: 0171 269 3213
Funds research into the prevention and cure of cancer.

INSTITUTE FOR COMPLEMENTARY MEDICINE

PO Box 194, London SE16 1QZ
Tel: 0171 237 5175
    Administers the British Register of Complementary Practitioners.

LYMPHOEDEMA SUPPORT NETWORK

St Luke's Crypt, Sydney Street, London SW3 6NH
Tel: 0171 351 4480
    Offers advice and support to sufferers of lymphoedema.

NATIONAL CANCER ALLIANCE

PO Box 579, Oxford OX4 1LB
Tel: 01865 793 566
    A membership organization that aims to ensure high-quality cancer treatment and care throughout the UK. It publishes a directory of cancer specialists.

NATIONAL FEDERATION OF SPIRITUAL HEALERS

Old Manor Farm Studio, Church Street, Sunbury on Thames, Middlesex, TW16 6RG
Tel: 0891 616 080
    Operates a national healer referral service.

VOLUNTARY EUTHANASIA SOCIETY

13 Prince of Wales Terrace, London W8 5PG
Tel: 0171 937 7770
    Can supply living wills.

UNITED STATES

ASSOCIATION OF COMMUNITY CANCER CENTERS

11600 Nebel Street, Suite 201, Rockville, MD 20852
Tel: 301-984-9496
    Provides a national forum for addressing the future of cancer care programs, including third party reimbursement, clinical research and quality care measures.

AMERICAN CANCER SOCIETY

1559 Clifton Road, NE, Atlanta, GA 30329
Tel: 1-800-ACS-2345 (1-800-227-2345) toll-free, or see the white pages of your local telephone directory
    A voluntary organization with local units offering many services and

activities all over the country.

CANCER CARE

1180 Avenue of the Americas, New York, NY 10036
Tel: 1-800-813-HOPE (1-800-813-4673) toll-free

A non-profit social service agency that provides a toll-free telephone counselling service to offer immediate psychological support to cancer patients and their families. It can also help with second opinions, dealing with the health care system, local community resources, financial assistance, pain management, access to entitlements and provide information on telephone support groups.

CANCER INFORMATION SERVICE

Tel: 1-800-4-CANCER (1-800-422-6237) toll-free; this connects callers with the office that serves their area

A program of the National Cancer Institute, offers a nationwide telephone service for cancer patients, friends, families and health care professionals. Staff can answer questions and send booklets about cancer. They may also know about local resources and services. Spanish-speaking staff are available.

PDQ (PHYSICIAN DATA QUERY)

Tel: Cancer Information Service (as above); or use the Cancerfax service, dialling 301-402-5874 from your fax machine

The National Cancer Institute's computerized listing of up-to-date and accurate information on the latest types of cancer treatments, research studies, clinical trials, new and promising cancer treatments, and organizations and doctors involved in caring for people with cancer.

NATIONAL COALITION OF CANCER SURVIVORSHIP (NCCS)

1010 Wayne Avenue, 5th floor, Silver Spring, MD 20910
Tel: 301-650-8868

Exists to enhance the quality of life for cancer survivors and to promote an understanding of cancer survivorship.

NATIONAL LYMPHEDEMA NETWORK

2211 Post Street, Suite 404, San Francisco, CA 94115
Tel: 800-541-3259

Provides information on the prevention and management of lymphedema.

FURTHER READING

These books are all worthwhile, but serve different purposes and some are much more technical than others. Browse or borrow before you buy!

Batt, Sharon *Patient No More: The Politics of Breast Cancer*, Scarlet Press, London, 1994

Benjamin, Harold H. PhD with Trubo, Richard, *From Victim to Victor*, Dell Publishing, New York, 1987

Disability Alliance *Disability Rights Handbook*, Disability Alliance, London, published annually

Farago, Robert *Hypnohealth*, Vermilion, London, 1995

National Coalition for Cancer Survivorship *An Almanac of Practical Resources for Cancer Survivors*, Consumers Union, Mount Vernon, New York, 1990

Ornstein, Robert and Sobel, David *The Healing Brain*, Macmillan, London, 1989

Rowe, Dorothy *Time is on Our Side*, Harper Collins, London, 1995

Speechley, Val and Rosenfield, Maxine *Cancer Information at Your Fingertips*, Class Publishing, London, 1995

Thomas, Dr Hilary and Sikora, Professor Karol *Cancer, A Positive Approach*, Thorsons, London, 1995

Tobias, Dr Jeffrey *Cancer: What Every Patient Needs to Know*, Bloomsbury, London, 1995

Woodham, Anne *HEA Guide to Complementary Medicine and Therapies*, Health Education Authority, 1994

INDEX